THE PSYCHODYNAMICS
OF STUTTERING

THE PSYCHODYNAMICS
OF STUTTERING

By

DOMINICK A. BARBARA, M.D., F.A.P.A.

Practicing Psychoanalyst
Associated with the American Institute for Psychoanalysis
Former Head of the Speech Department
Karen Horney Clinic
New York, New York

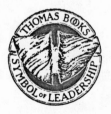

CHARLES C THOMAS • PUBLISHER
Springfield • Illinois • U.S.A.

Published and Distributed Throughout the World by
CHARLES C THOMAS • PUBLISHER
2600 South First Street
Springfield, Illinois 62717, U.S.A.

© *1982 by* CHARLES C THOMAS • PUBLISHER
ISBN 0-398-04714-6
Library of Congress Catalog Card Number: 82-5570

*With THOMAS BOOKS careful attention is given to all details of
manufacturing and design. It is the Publisher's desire to present books that are
satisfactory as to their physical qualities and artistic possibilities and
appropriate for their particular use. THOMAS BOOKS will be true to those
laws of quality that assure a good name and good will.*

Printed in the United States of America
I-R5-1

Library of Congress Cataloging in Publication Data

Barbara, Dominick A.
  The psychodynamics of stuttering.

  Bibliography: p.
  Includes index.
  1. Stuttering—Psychological aspects. 2. Stuttering—Treatment. I. Title. [DNLM: 1. Stuttering—Psychology. WM
475 B229p]
RC424.B216   616.85'54   82-5570
ISBN 0-398-04714-6   AACR2

PREFACE

ALTHOUGH volumes have been written on the cause and effect of stuttering, little has been compiled concerning the understanding and therapy of the problem from a holistic viewpoint. Stuttering can no longer be seen primarily as a vocal problem due to difficulty in articulation or breathing. This problem is much more complex and concerns the whole person, for the function of speech is not only to express ideas, but to adjust us to other people. Stuttering occurs when these functions fail to operate smoothly, as the stutterer anxiously attempts to restore his psychic balance.

The symptom is so dramatic and so obviously troublesome that it is a temptation to anyone working with stutterers to try to do something about the symptom, whereas the relief of the underlying difficulty is the only thing that can give eventual and permanent relief.

Much of the material in this volume has been extracted and revised from my previous writings on stuttering over the past twenty-five years. An attempt has been made to give a simple and concise presentation with the hope in mind that speech therapists can utilize my concepts in their own therapy with stutterers.

Finally, a recommendation is made that a team approach to the problems of stuttering be studied and implemented, joining together the skills and orientation of both the speech therapist and the psychotherapist.

D.A.B.

CONTENTS

OTHER BOOKS BY THE AUTHOR

STUTTERING: A Psychodynamic Approach to Its Understanding and
    Treatment
YOUR SPEECH REVEALS YOUR PERSONALITY (3rd Printing)
THE ART OF LISTENING (4th Printing)
LOVING AND MAKING LOVE
THE HEALTHY MIND IN COMMUNION AND COMMUNICATION
QUESTIONS AND ANSWERS ON STUTTERING
Editor: PSYCHOLOGICAL AND PSYCHIATRIC ASPECTS OF SPEECH
    AND HEARING
Editor: THE PSYCHOTHERAPY OF STUTTERING
Editor: NEW DIRECTIONS IN STUTTERING

THE PSYCHODYNAMICS
OF STUTTERING

Chapter 1

STUTTERING: SPEECH PROBLEM
OR EMOTIONAL DISORDER?

M OST speech pathologists in general think of stuttering as one kind of speech disorder, and so they accept without question the assertion that stuttering should be treated by themselves or by some others of their professional colleagues.

The speech therapist maintains that an inability to produce a particular sound or word can be traced to some part of the vocal mechanism, most likely the laryngeal mechanism, and stuttering therefore can be traced to some part of the vocal mechanism that is operating in a deviate way or in a combination of the various parts of the vocal mechanism acting deviately together. From this viewpoint, in short, stuttering is a disorganization of the vocal mechanism. The speech therapists may disagree among themselves as to the cause of the disorganization of the vocal mechanism that produces stuttering, but they agree that the vocal mechanism is the main area of the focus of treatment.

From the opposite viewpoint we find the psychotherapist who classes stuttering in the general category of symptoms of emotional disturbance. Within this body of opinion, two main positions are identifiable. The first asserts that the emotional disturbance is the cause of the stuttering. The second maintains that the reverse situation holds and that the emotional disturbance is the result of the frustrations and failures in interpersonal relationships, which the stutterer's pattern of nonfluent speech imposes upon him.

The first position, that stuttering is one of the ways in which

3

an emotional disturbance may exhibit itself, has been labeled the neurotic theory of stuttering. It is the one that I have written about so extensively over the years and the one that a good many speech pathologists, and most psychiatrists, psychologists, and social workers have endorsed.

Although some speech pathologists have had reservations about the neurotic explanation of stuttering, most of them agree, however, that a pattern of emotional disturbances exists in all, or most, stutterers. *The stutterer stutters not with his mouth alone, but with his whole body*—his speech, his feelings, and his relationships to himself and to others!

In my opinion, stuttering is primarily due to the anxiety of the stutterer in coping with the world he lives in and in his chaotic attempts to adjust to other people. Whether the origins of stuttering are basically emotional or whether stuttering in itself creates emotional disturbances is not in itself crucial. What is essential and what needs to be stressed again and again is that the treatment of the stutterer should consist not only of vocal exercises and suggestions, but the treatment of the whole person.

The symptom is so dramatic and so obviously troublesome that it is a temptation to anyone working with stutterers to try to do something about the symptom, whereas the relief of the underlying difficulty is also imperative to give eventual and permanent relief.

In the realm of speech disorders, stuttering plays a most prevalent and important role. It is a highly complex syndrome with multiple etiology, combining genogenic, morphogenic, chemogenic, neurogenic, psychogenic, and socio-environmental factors. Only by approaching it from a holistic viewpoint, with an emphasis on the total organism, can we hope to understand its nature and treatment.

Although many speech pathologists may have reservations about the emotional explanation of stuttering, they do most often agree that a pattern of emotional disturbances exists in all, or most, stutterers. They account for it most as a consequence of social experiences involving communication in which stuttering patterns have existed over a long period of time. These same speech pathologists contend that since we live in a society where verbal communication is overvalued, stuttering becomes seen as a deficiency, an impediment. The stutterer himself, with all his exaggerated sensitivities, reacts to these social values with a sense of inferiority, guilt, and helplessness. He feels that if he didn't stutter he would be a better and a more successfully functioning individual and more acceptable to himself and others.

It is my opinion that many theoreticians approaching stuttering from a psychological basis have met with pitfalls because of adherence to a genetic approach, with overemphasis on cause and effect concomitants. When one takes into account the tremendous number of stutterers in our present society, it is not difficult to understand why a study project to its etiology can assume boundless proportions. A statistical cross section pertaining to quantitative factors having common denominations in this one specific problem seems to me to have little relative value. Another shortcoming in the field of theoretical investigation of stuttering has been in approaching it from a mechanistic-evolutionistic viewpoint rather than from a dynamic orientation. This sort of thinking presupposes that symptom reactions are conditioned entirely by something in the past, and that as a result they persist in the present in the pattern of original development. This view also stresses the importance of constitutional origins in practically all forms of disease entities. Though I do affirm that constitution is a relatively fixed quantity that plays a role of some importance in individual development, it is a small factor when compared to the resultant impact of interpersonal experiences on the same person.

Regardless of the etiology of stuttering, however, the fact remains that the confirmed stutterer presents a picture of an insecure, chronically anxious, highly excitable, emotionally immature person in most social situations and a morbidly fearful person in speech situations. It is this weakened personality as it presents itself at the time of treatment that necessitates changing, rather than the formulation of involved theories regarding its etiology. It is essential that one work with the stutterer as he presents himself in the present to probe deeper into his past for cause-effect equivalents.

Stuttering involves the whole personality, which comprises emotion, intellect, and volition. The stutterer has acquired his difficulty as he has come to possess any of his other mental acquisitions and emotional reaction tendencies. One can no more localize it than he can localize these. Hence the error and the false hope involved in thinking that we can "uproot," "break up from within," or "cast out" this disorder of speech with the same sort of dispatch with which a surgeon can remedy a distorted limb or remove a diseased tonsil. He who encourages the spread of this conception of stuttering is, therefore, not only incorrectly oriented scientifically, but is likely to be of social disservice by bolstering popular faith in shortcut cures.

The treatment of stuttering from a psychological viewpoint is primarily an individual process and cannot be thought of in terms of masses. The stutterer is not a cripple of society, and to think of him as such tends to overstress the social impact of the problem. To grant him special privileges in his environment tends only to increase his basic claims on life because he may then feel that as a stutterer, he is entitled to these privileges. This implied attitude of feeling socially inferior to others may engender his associated feeling of helplessness and inadequacy, leading all the more to a robbing of self-growth, self-respect, and responsibility for one's self.

A therapeutic approach has to take into account both intrapsychic and interpersonal factors in order to help the stutterer understand the nature of his speech problem and its conflicting tendencies. Only as he can feel how bound and driven he is by his own stuttering and its emotional entanglements, will he be able to face himself. Finally, the more he is able to face himself as an equal, responsible, and self-perpetuating unit of society, the more courage he will have to give up his speech impediment and relate to others with assertiveness and conviction. To accomplish this, the emphasis must be placed not only on his deviated speech but on the underlying forces that drive him to stutter; and, finally, on the feelings, attitudes, and responses in the crucial speaking situation.

An approach to stuttering exclusively from a psychological viewpoint, that of improving his emotional health, is likely to be inadequate if the nonfluent patterns of speech persist. The nonfluent speech in the eyes of the stutterer constitutes the core of his problem and the one in which he insists on being helped. This could be a blocking stone in the therapeutic process and one in which the help of a speech therapist may be needed.

Some time ago I edited a book entitled *The Psychotherapy of Stuttering* in which Doctor Jesse J. Villarreal wrote an excellent and provocative chapter, "The Role of the Speech Pathologist in Psychotherapy." To quote extensively from his writings, Doctor Villarreal states—

> The term 'team approach' is used with increasing frequency to describe therapeutic programs in which a number of specializations work together cooperatively in a complicated rehabilitation process. What is being recommended here is a team approach for the problems of stuttering, an approach in which the therapy team includes the skills and orientation of a speech therapist and the skills and orientation of a psychotherapist.
>
> It should be pointed out that what is being insisted upon here is not that the union lines between the speech pathologist and the psychotherapist be rigorously preserved, and that penalties be invoked when the one threatens to cross over into the domain of the other. There is nothing inherent in the situation that makes it impossible for a single person to possess and to employ whatever special talents may be peculiar either to the speech pathologist or the psychotherapist. Quite a few individuals think they possess, and a somewhat smaller number can demonstrate by the programs of training they have followed that they do possess, the skills of both speech pathology and psychotherapy. There are persons who are Fellows of the American Speech and Hearing Association or holders of a medical degree with specialization in psychiatry, or both!
>
> What is being said is that persons with this breadth of professional training are rare, and are not ever likely to be numerous, and are certain to be far less numerous than is needed for the treatment of stuttering. It follows, then, that if an adequate program of therapy for stutterers will generally require the special talents both of the speech pathologist and the psychotherapist, most of the practitioners in either field will be inadequately prepared to perform both functions well, and the team approach is called for.
>
> A therapy program along the lines that have been described is approximated, although perhaps not exploited to the fullest possible extent, in a number of programs already in existence. These programs possess all, or most, of the following characteristics:
>
> 1. Therapy for the problem of stuttering is viewed as a joint activity of a therapy team that includes a speech pathologist and a clinical psychologist or psychiatrist.

2. The diagnostic examination of the stutterer includes attention to the vocal-mechanism centered aspects, superintended by a speech pathologist, and attention to the emotional health of the stutterer, superintended by a clinical psychologist. Generally, the stutterer will be administered a battery of such tests as the clinical psychologist has available, particularly projective tests, that are held to be capable of throwing light on the state of emotional health of a person.

3. There will be abundant opportunities for interaction by the two therapies, with consultations at the diagnostic level, joint plannings of therapy activities, and assessment that is broad enough to include evidences of speech fluency and evidences of emotional health as well.

A program of the kind described here, obviously is not always to be had wherever stutterers are treated at present. For the speech clinic located in a university or college, a beginning has, in a number of instances, been made in the growing recognition that an adequately staffed speech clinic will include a person possessing the special skills of the clinical psychologist.

In brief summary at this point, we may conclude—

1. Stuttering must be seen as a holistic syndrome involving both a deviate way of operating the vocal mechanism and a complexity of emotional intricacies.

2. Working with the emotional disturbance is most essential to the ultimate therapeutic result. Whether this emotional disturbance is viewed as the basic cause of stuttering or the inevitable result of it is not the prime criteria for positive results. What is important is that it is there and needs attention.

3. At the same time it must be recognized that where emotional changes occur and the speech deviation persists, the intervention by a speech pathologist is essential to assist in working with those kinds of disorganization that require modifications in the activity of the vocal mechanism.

4. Finally, it is therefore necessary and ideal that for the most adequate treatment of stuttering (here I concur wholeheartedly with Doctor Villarreal), a therapy team with both the skills of the speech pathologist and those of the psychotherapist should be utilized. For this therapy team to function efficiently there should be a familiarity by each specialty of the other. Although the therapeutic approach may not be suitable for all existing speech therapists and psychotherapists, it is certainly an ideal goal to work towards.

A combined therapeutic approach to stuttering may not be suited for all speech therapists or psychotherapists who adhere blindly to their own professions. Both can and should learn from each other's experiences and knowledge, in the spirit of cooperation and familiarity. The speech therapist will need to be willing to obtain some background and clinical experience in the psychodynamics of stuttering. The converse is equally true. That psychotherapist will be most useful as a member of the team approach whose academic and clinical experience has included a substantial knowledge and acquaintance with speech and hearing problems and with stuttering in particular. The ideal, therefore, is a cooperative team approach with two kinds of disciplines used jointly and acting in concert. The trend has already begun, and it is my sincere hope, after working thirty-five years with stutterers, that this will prove to give successful and lasting results. The stutterer will as a result of this joint approach not only give up his stuttering, but be able to be a more fulfilled and productive human being. It is with this intent in mind that I am writing this book. As a psychotherapist I will elaborate on the psychodynamics of stuttering and conclude with some ideas of mine on the combined therapeutic approach.

Chapter 2

BASIC DYNAMICS IN THE
DEVELOPMENT OF STUTTERING

EARLY CHILDHOOD AND PARENTAL
INFLUENCES IN STUTTERING

THE soil from which the individual who stutters grows and develops is similar in nature to that in other forms of psychosomatic disorders. It differs mainly in regard to the quality and degree of the individual responses and experiences to the particular environmental background.

In order to describe unhealthy growth, we must begin with an understanding of what is healthy and what are the prerequisites for healthy development. Although there are essential similarities in the growth patterns of individuals, no two children, even those in the same family constellation, are alike, either in themselves or in the way that they move through this sequence of development. Each child, when born, has his own moods, temperaments, potentialities, gifts, and his own particular capacities. In the same context, each individual child has his own physical, mental, and emotional attributes. A child afflicted at birth with some organic defect will most likely have a greater difficulty in adjusting and progressing through the periods of development than a more fortunate physically healthy one. In addition, cultural and economic factors at the time of birth also play an important role in the future developmental growth of the particular individual.

Individuals inherently tend toward self-realization and constructive individual growth. Given the chance and a more or less healthy soil, a child can grow to become apparently normal and

10

fulfill his growth possibilities. Basically the soil must contain a feeling of genuine warmth, love, and respect. A child needs to feel that his environment is one in which he is wanted, loved, and needed and one in which there is a sense of belonging. If this feeling is lacking, then a state of emotional stirring, which is felt as difficult to understand or accept, is generated in the child. He may thus begin to be rendered weak, insecure, and shaky. This can easily be the focal point around which the origin of his difficulties, with increasing further frustrations and disappointments, begin to be felt.

The reason why a child does not receive adequate love and warmth at this stage of development may lie in the parents' incapacity to convey it because of their own problems. This may be expressed either openly in the form of hostility toward an unwanted child, revealed by the parents' detached, disinterested, and aloof attitude, or camouflaged in the form of an oversolicitude or the self-sacrificing attitude of an "ideal" mother.

The following are brief illustrations of various combinations of parental settings in stutter-type environments.

Case 1

Johnny's family on both sides were of German-Polish descent, middle class. He is an only child born through a forced marriage due to an illegitimate pregnancy. His mother is a large, heavyset, domineering, and perfectionistic individual. In her own family constellation she played a minor role, being constantly oppressed and pushed into the background by her own mother and older sister, who was the family favorite. Johnny's father played a detached, aloof, and indifferent role, succumbing many times to his wife's demands in order to avoid too many arguments or friction. As a boy, Johnny was in constant fear of being punished for not being able to live up to his mother's absolute and perfectionistic demands. She exposed him to a domineering form of overprotection, as she dictated and charted every possible move he took. Onset of stuttering began at the age of nine.

Case 2

Robert was born in New York in 1912. Both sides of the family were of Russian-Jewish descent and of the middle class. His

mother is described as a small, aggressive, domineering, and controlling individual who assumed the dominant role in her own marriage. In her own family constellation, however, she played a minute role, being the only girl of a family of four siblings. In this
family setting of hers, she felt as though she had to constantly
assert herself in order to survive. She is further described as being
extremely touchy, sensitive, suspicious, exploitative, and living
under false pretenses of being lovable, honest, and sincere. Robert's
father is described as being a detached, shy, withdrawn, and retir-
ing person who had little time for himself or his children. Toward
him, his wife was constantly complaining, nagging, and belittling.
After constant quarrels and bitter friction, Robert's father desert-
ed his family and his whereabouts were unknown. This left his
wife with all the more justification to feel embittered and abused.
She was now compelled to go to work, and into the household
came her own mother, who complicated the situation all the more.
As a child, Robert was sickly and fragile. His mother felt guilty
as a result of this and exposed him to a morbid form of overprotection. She constantly watched over him, showered him with
gifts, embraced him affectionately whenever he conformed to her
expectations, yet raged when he rebelled. She accompanied him
to and from school, chose his friends, and was constantly in fear
that he would hurt himself or get sick. Robert was rarely permitted to go out to play with the other children and was not allowed
to partake in vigorous competitive sports. His mother would rule
him with an iron hand, yet at times shower him with gifts, over-
affection, and false love. As a result of this constant ambivalence
of emotion, Robert felt persistent confusion, doubt, and apprehension. Stuttering began at the age of seven.

Case 3

Tony was born in a poorer Italian section of Brooklyn in
1927. Both parents were Italian, born in Palermo, who had mi-
grated to this country because of social and economic goals. Tony
was the only boy in a family of five older sisters. There were eight
pregnancies in all, two of them ending in miscarriages. Tony's
father felt angered and hostile each time his wife gave birth to a
female child. He would rage at her for her incapacity to bear

worthwhile children and felt insignificant as a male in the eyes of his relatives and neighbors. He is further described as being aggressive, domineering, and controlling and as an arrogant, vindictive tyrant. Because of his own cultural background he strongly held to the dogma of male superiority. When Tony was born, his father shut his barber shop for a week, and the home became a temple of worship and festivity. His "Christ-like" son had been born and no longer had he to hang his head in shame and humiliation. Tony's mother, on the other hand, is described as being self-sacrificing, oversolicitous, and martyr-like in her suffering role. Tony's life had been charted and dictated ever since his birth. Because of the tremendous social and intellectual prestige accorded the professional man in this sort of cultural background, he was to become a successful doctor, lawyer, or dentist. The intense pressure of the unattainable goals forced upon Tony from an early age resulted in his beginning to stutter at the age of eight.

Case 4

Carmine was also born in a poorer section of Brooklyn in 1926. His parents were of Italian-Irish descent and of the middle class. The family environment was one of constant arguments and friction over money matters, in-laws, and religious issues. The father was a severe stutterer who drank habitually in the presence of his son. During his wife's second pregnancy, he brutally kicked her abdomen, causing her to abort. When Carmine was four years old, his father was killed in a street brawl during a drinking spree. Following this unfortunate event, Carmine's mother began to center all her energies and resources toward living vicariously through her son. She overprotected him and held him close to her "apron strings." She went to work, boarded him with a neighbor of hers, and made up her mind never to marry again. She prayed and believed that her son would magically give her everything she wished for and of which she had been so cruelly and unjustly deprived. Carmine was her "baby," her only salvation toward peace and tranquility. She guarded her precious possession with every ounce of her strength and watched him grow with fear, apprehension, and selfish protectiveness. He started to stutter at the age of six.

A child's position in a family unit can be made to be predominant, unique, special, or different in itself from most other healthy children's environment. Factors that lead to this sort of a unique yet precarious position result from some of the following basic sources:

1. The child predisposed to stuttering is usually an only child in a family unit. This may come about as a definite choice in a selfish, sacrificing mother or realistically following a long period of absence of pregnancy as a result of several abortions and miscarriages. It can be the result of separation, divorce, or of the immediate death of one of the parents, usually the father. At other times, economic factors may compel the mother to go to work, with the ensuing result that a choice is made to have no additional children.

2. The stuttering child's position can become predominant as a result of his being the only male child in a family of two or more other females. Here we find that the added attentions, stresses, and demands are placed immediately upon him because of his unique position.

3. A third and concluding source, I feel, arises from definite, deeply imbedded traditional cultural factors found in some parents of children who stutter. Many of these children are from families of minority groups—Italians, Jews, Negroes, Poles, etc.—where the cultural milieu gives importance to the special meaning of the male preference, the first son, or the firstborn. Stress is also placed on the social importance of male superiority to female inferiority. In the home, the male is generally looked up to as the master, the sole provider, the basic stronghold of the relationship, while the female usually takes the back seat in the sense of being the weaker sex. A male child born into a milieu of this sort, as can be seen, is bound to succumb to the pressing demands of its impossible heights and to feel driven and torn.

THE ONSET OF STUTTERING

The average age at which children usually begin to stutter is about two years, rarely after the age of nine. It is at about this age that the average child begins to show enough meaning to his speech to have his parents pay attention to what he is saying and how he is saying it.

Free-flowing and spontaneous speech in a child is obtained mostly in an environment of parental warmth and freedom and one in which the child feels accepted. Hesitancies in talking, however, first begin to express themselves in response to a parental setting of prohibitions and restitutions. This nonfluent speech and hesitancy in younger children may be normal to some degree, yet tense, overworried, and perfectionistic parents may tend to look to this as stuttering. Once the child has been labeled as a stutterer, his position again becomes unique, in that there is set in motion a chain reaction of worries, anxieties, and preoccupations, which gravely perturbs both child and parent.

A child's hesitancies in speech are further aggravated in parent-child situations that interfere with the normal expression of thought, feeling, and action. In a home in which there is overemphasis on perfectionistic standards and regimes, there may well be present attitudes conducive to disapproval of nonfluent speech. A perfectionistic parent may compel his child to speak perfectly, clearly, and loudly. If the child talks slowly, words are practically taken out of his mouth or interpreted for him. He may be constantly criticized for hesitating before starting to speak, and when he finally does, for not saying the right words in the first place. He is taught to feel that words must be carefully chosen and that he must articulate clearly and master his communications. He must not falter or hesitate too long and must be brief about what he has to say and yet at the same time be prepared to say whatever may be expected of him at any time. Some perfectionistic parents may even go so far as to suggest other methods of talking that they feel will be better or easier for the child. These latter suggestions may include showing the child how to inhale before speaking and exhale afterward, to substitute other words for the more difficult ones whenever a hesitancy may occur, or to exercise willpower and to push speech, even though the child may feel fatigued or excited. Parents of this sort will generally lose their own patience in the use of some of these rigid compulsions of theirs and finally resort to some form of punishment, ridicule, or even sadistic embarrassment of the child in the presence of others.

The overprotective parent makes as many demands and expectations in her child's beginning speech development as the perfectionistic one, though here the attitudes are usually camouflaged
with a facade of overconcern, worry, and a persistent state of pre-
occupation. The child, because of the overemphasis on being pro-
tected, is made to feel dependent upon his parent for constant
approval, praise, and recognition each time he expresses himself.
He is taught to develop *shoulds* in what he is supposed to say, each
time he opens his mouth. His language in words is not experienced
as being his own, but as coming from the outside, usually identified with his overprotective and dominant mother. He learns to
mimic and imitate his mother in almost every way: "Mommy says
don't do this, say this, eat this, watch out, be careful," etc. His
speech begins to be felt as alien to him, rigid in nature, compulsive, hesitating, and filled with doubts and apprehensions. When
he talks, he is driven to adhere to strict parental activities concerning what to say, how to say it, and when to say it. Most overprotective parents feel that their children should be "seen but not
heard." They should never intrude when Mommy is talking,
should have good manners, and should keep absolutely quiet when
others are present. These same parents may listen quite attentively
to their children when they feel it necessary, yet show very little
consistent real interest or attention when needed. A child in such
a prohibitive environment develops a fear and apprehension of
talking. He becomes afraid of what will happen to him if he should
talk at the wrong time or say something that may suddenly slip
out and not meet with his mother's approval. He feels generally
guilty each time he speaks in the presence of a parent of this
sort and makes every possible attempt to control his thoughts and
to measure his words. Should he then hesitate or have difficulty
in talking, which is quite likely, under such emotional stress he
becomes all the more "thrown out of emotional gear" by the worrisome and anxious reactions of his parents. We thus see, as has already been mentioned, the setting into motion of a vicious circle
of chain reactions of traumatic consequence to the child's further
speech developments.

Beginning speech is normally quite nonfluent. The average
child aged two to six years old repeats about forty-five times per

thousand words. He repeats sounds, or parts of words, *like th- th-this*; or whole words, *like like like this*; or phrases, *like this like this like this*. Besides, he engages in various other types of hesitancies, stallings, *ums, ahs*, etc. All this is perfectly normal. Some children are more hesitant and repetitious than others (there are individual differences in everything), but no child so far studied has been found to be perfectly fluent by any means.

In most homes, particularly those in which no one has had any personal experience with stuttering, the normal nonfluency of beginning speech is almost completely disregarded. Most parents are surprised to learn that the average youngster repeats forty-five times per thousand words; they had not noticed or do not remember that their own children did any repeating to speak of. About 99 percent of our children are permitted to develop speech, with all its normal nonfluencies, without being made self-conscious about it by parents who are overly concerned and perfectionistic. The basic question is not so much what causes some children to stutter, but rather what causes an occasional parent to cultivate the attitudes and policies that tend to make for stuttering in the child.

The reasons for the onset of stuttering are not to be sought within the child or even in the way he speaks, but inside his parents' head, or, rather, in the parents' attitudes and reactions to the way the child speaks. The point not to be missed is that any child speaks with enough nonfluency to be worried about and diagnosed as stuttering provided his parents are prepared, by their conditioned attitudes, beliefs, and standards, to worry enough and to see simple repetitions and hesitancies as danger signals. Parents differ amazingly in this general respect. Any one parent, moreover, fluctuates with regard to the way he evaluates and reacts to the speech of any one of his children or of his two or more different children. Circumstances vary, competing sources of concern shift about, distractions of all sorts arise and subside, and the total impression made by a child at one time differs markedly, for changing and complex reasons, from the impressions made by the same child on the same parent at another time. What may be totally unnoticed one day may be suddenly perceived as stuttering the next and disregarded again a week later.

The onset of stuttering in childhood may be precipitated by any experience that in an emotionally inadequate child generates anxiety and fear. Such traumatic experiences are fright, accident, illness, operations, forcible conversion from left- to right-handedness, or a tense and worrisome home environment. The element of fright as a situational traumatic experience plays the most prevalent role. The most common experiences of this type are being frightened by the dark or lightning, receiving a severe punishment at the hands of a domineering and stern parent; being frightened by a dog or some other animal; being chased or mobbed by a gang of tough boys; being yelled at by an angered person; being thrown into water for the first time; and being caught in the act of masturbation by a parent.

The following examples are illustrations of some cases of adult stuttering—individuals whom I've studied, with known precipitating factors beginning in early childhood.

Case 1

L.H., an only child, was closely attached to his mother, who overprotected him and held him very close to her "apron strings." During his early childhood, she directed his mode of living and shook his feelings of security. She constantly spoke to him of the dangers and cruelties of the outside world and forbade him to associate with the rest of the boys in the neighborhood. He presented a history of nail-biting, enuresis at the age of nine, and frequent nightmares of a terrifying nature. At the age of six, after much persuasion, he went along with a group of his playmates to a nearby vacant building, which his mother had constantly warned him not to visit, because it was supposed to be haunted. As he entered the building, one of the older boys decided to play a prank on him by pushing him through a doorway and running away with the rest of the group. This incident of being isolated in a forbidden spot was of a frightening nature, and subsequently he stuttered.

Case 2

N.H., a thirty-five-year-old male, was the product of a domineering, stern, and rigid mother and an alcoholic father, who had little time to spend with his children. The family environment was one of constant friction and quarrels. At an early age he was subject to nail-biting, temper tantrums, and nightmares of being beaten up. His eldest brother was his constant and only companion and the one in whom he confided and whom he respected. At the age of eight while chasing his brother through the streets while playing, he saw his brother being struck by a truck and instantly killed. Involuntarily following this tremendous psychic shock he began to stutter.

Case 3

R.B., a fifty-year-old female, was dominated most of her life by a tyrannical and intolerant father who punished her frequently. When she was five, she remembers that her mother suddenly became psychotic and was confined to a mental institution. During her early childhood, she was subjected to horrifying nightmares of being chased by weird animals who would awaken her and cause her to have nocturnal crying spells. At the age of seven she was frightened by a large dog and subsequently began to stutter.

Case 4

S.R., a twenty-year-old male, was the only child of parents who were drug addicts. The father was a severe stutterer, and frequently, when he became angered, would beat his wife in the presence of his son. The mother later took to alcohol, and when the boy first entered school, he was shy, reclusive, and insecure. Whenever he was about to be called upon to speak in class, he would become afraid and break out into a complete sweat. His lips would tremble and he couldn't speak for some time. He had been a chronic nail-biter up to the age of fifteen, and there is a history of being a sleepwalker in earlier years. At the age of seven, he was forced, upon the insistence of his father, to undergo a tonsillectomy. The severe fright and shock sustained during this incident were followed by stuttering.

Case 5

D.S., an eighteen-year-old male, went swimming at the age of eight against his mother's wishes. While attempting to dive, he slipped and struck his skull against a plank, receiving a slight injury to his forehead. He was not unconscious, but temporarily shocked and frightened. This frightening experience, plus the anticipation of being punished by the mother, was alleged to have caused his stuttering.

Case 6

A.D., a thirty-three-year-old male, was left handed since birth. Both parents were described as being vigorous, intolerant, and demanding. There is a history of a brother and a maternal cousin who stuttered. There was a constant fear of not meeting his parents' demands and of receiving some form of punishment in consequence. As a child he wet the bed and had frequent nightmares of falling off tall buildings or of floating off into space, without being able to come back to earth. At the age of five, he was forcibly threatened to be converted from left- to right-handedness, and subsequently stuttered.

Case 7

T.R., an eighteen-year-old male, began to stutter at the age of nine, following an attack of encephalitis lethargica. His family history denoted a highly neurotic, temperamental, high-strung, and worrisome mother. The father died of an unknown cause when the boy was six years old. A maternal aunt stuttered and later became psychotic. During the entire course of illness, the mother remained constantly at his bedside, sobbed, cried, and prayed continually for his recovery. He has been a chronic nail-biter and wet the bed until the age of twelve.

The above case illustrations are not meant to be examples of cause-effect relationships in stuttering. They have been cited to illustrate conditions in which emotionally disturbed children can be prone to feel threatened in the face of overwhelming anxiety-provoking situations and as a result give expression to their fear in the speaking situation.

Stuttering as a psychosomatic disturbance is only a symptom of emotional conflict. A child rendered basically helpless, insecure, and afraid is driven toward safety and some degree of pseudo harmony. Since these same trends are compulsive, inappropriate, and contradictory in nature, they are bound to fail in the face of the slightest threatening situation. With additional frustrations and disturbances to his neurotic status quo, the emotionally weakened child is faced with the full awareness of his precarious position and as a result is in a state of continual fear, anxiety, and hostility.

As the stuttering child struggles to combat his inner conflicts, he has too little awareness of what to do or where to turn, in order to release himself from his emotional entanglements. He feels imprisoned by his own problems, and as he makes spasmodic attempts toward some form of integration, he becomes even more frustrated, anxious, and panic-stricken. A vicious circle is created, with too little peace or visible restoration, leading finally to feelings of misery, hopelessness, and inertia.

In our particular culture, language is considered the chief medium of communication. Through it we express our opinions, feelings, attitudes, and actions. The earliest conflicts of a child are expressed in his communications, both socially and verbally, to his parents and to the outside world about him. Where other children can pass through the primary stages of communication and early development less afflicted, the stutterer, because of his emotionally crippled position, is much more prone to anxiety.

To summarize, the child who tends toward developing stuttering stems from the following possible sources: (1) Disturbed parental and environmental factors at an early age cause him to become weakened and to generate basic anxiety with its accompanying feelings of helplessness and hostility; (2) as a result of the early age at which these threatening sources begin, the child, because of his emotionally weakened condition, is unable to organize enough forces together to restore order to his disorganized state; (3) as a form of safety and protection to his already crippled personality, unhealthy trends are developed, which, because of their contradictory nature, create further conflicts; (4) since language is the chief medium of communication at this time, it is also the area that first tends to disorganize when the protective structures of the organism are threatened and as a result gives experience to anxiety; (5) the speaking situation, which is normally used to convey an idea, express a feeling, or ask a question, now becomes converted into a self-assertive, self-conscious act in an environment that gives rise to emotions of hostility and fear. Simple social situations in which speech is required unconsciously become testing grounds for possible social combat. The hesitation that results from the conflict between the rational impulse to speak and the irrational fear of speaking becomes crystallized as stuttering. Psychologically the process is no different from the occasional stuttering of the normal child or adult. The difference is only quantitative. A vicious cycle is soon established. Speech is an instrument for the mastery of the environment, as it is through speech that the child acquires knowledge and experience and tells of his need for affection and reassurance. As the need for mastery is urgent and as every effort in this direction is rendered ineffectual by fear and hesitation, more efforts are made and more anxiety produced. (6) At first the child, except for the expression of some subjective feelings of tension, awkwardness, or slight muscular incoordination, is unaware of the seriousness of his stuttering condition. However, the added stresses, fears, threats, and apprehensions of his anxious parents tend to make the child fix his attention even more on the speaking situation. The child is made to feel that when he speaks he is not perfect and that he is different from others and somewhat of a weird creature in society. As a result, he begins to feel inferior to other children, peculiar, and self-conscious. Finally, when this same child enters school, the added stress and the particular competitive atmosphere of this environment further cripple his personality. Added emphasis is placed on the dangers and threats of the speaking situation. Speech that is ordinarily not conscious now becomes conscious and identified with fears of both social rejection and the fear of stuttering. (7) In the confirmed or adult stutterer, there is a further development of the weakened structure, with additional complex attempts at solutions and with the use of stuttering as a means of externalizing conflict. Finally, all of this chaos and insecurity becomes openly expressed implicitly in the speaking situation.

Chapter 3

THE FURTHER DEVELOPMENT OF
THE ADULT STUTTERER'S PERSONALITY

THE person who stutters feels at most times apart and different from others in his society. He may feel that although others also have difficulties in life, they can cope with them and live much more easily with their problems. He feels more permanently crippled than others because of the fact that he cannot hide or conceal his speech difficulty. Therefore he is the constant target of their embarrassment, ridicule, and disapproval. He may rationalize to the effect that persons with migraine headaches, asthma, stomach ulcers, etc. suffer; however, they can still keep their troubles to themselves and go on living, while he, being unable to speak fluently, has the added burden of social criticism and judgment. As a result he may feel that the world should provide him special services and privileges and entitle him to a position in life, a job suitable to his speech incapacity. He wants a society that will make allowances for his stuttering, yet at the same time not make it appear too obvious that he is crippled. Along with these notions he may feel embittered and blame his particular culture, with its telephones, dictaphones, and other means of verbal communication. Since he fears and feels these same objects as threats to his protective shield, he may experience himself as a victim of this society and expect all the more due special privileges and rights.

He further feels that others should take over for him in those speaking situations where he might encounter some difficulty. Others should answer the telephone for him, make requests for him, give him exact information, and pay him absolute attention whenever he talks. He feels these are due since he then does not have to go through the bother and inconvenience of repeating himself. The reasoning here is that "since you know that I stutter in these particular situations, you should understand me perfectly well the first time and help me to avoid further embarrassment and ridicule."

Though he may feel legitimately justified in demanding special privileges of others, he is at the same time extremely sensitive to any form of criticism, doubting, or questioning of himself. Others should never pinpoint him into giving exact responses or concrete facts when conversing with him. Since he has a dire need to be right and feels trapped and coerced in exacting situations, he stutters easily in these particular threatening circumstances. Here again he distorts the realities by resorting to abused feelings and the claim that others, knowing how he suffers in these particular situations, should be easy on him and give him enough latitude in which to maneuver at all times. People should not ask him boldly or directly such exacting questions as "What is your name and address?," "How can I get to such and such an address?," etc. Questions that are asked of him should be absolutely clear and concise and should necessitate no more than one- or two-word answers. There should not be the need for elaborate or detailed explanations or discussions.

When he begins to speak, he feels entitled to absolute attention and the fullest of interest on the part of his listeners. Since he stutters, he feels that he has to weigh carefully his words before talking, and as a result what he says is of the utmost value. He should not have to repeat himself. People should be considerate and not interrupt him when he is speaking. As he speaks, others should not look away, yawn, or appear in any way distracted. When they call him by telephone, they should realize that he stutters, speak to him softly, and not become annoyed or harsh should he have difficulty. He should never be called on to testify in court, read in class, make reports to a group, or be held to specific reading situations. Others should take over these responsibilities for him, since he feels they have no difficulties in these areas. Little does he know, or want to know, that many other people have serious difficulties when speaking, although their conflicts may not necessarily be expressed in the form of stuttering. He feels that he should be excused at these times. Yet he becomes indignant and feels abused when he loses out in getting the credit of the praise involved in such endeavors.

In competitive situations, though basically aggressive, the person who stutters feels inclined to lean over backward and to allow others to take the initiative. Again, since he stutters, he demands that others should make things easy for him. Since pressures cause him to stutter, he expects others to understand his sensitive position and to place few obstacles or difficulties in his path. Though severely harsh and critical of others' shortcomings, he feels that he should be understood and respected at all times. When he stutters, he magically wishes and demands others to ease his threatened position, yet not to expose the fact that he himself is having difficulty in speaking. Others should substitute for him in crucial spots, do the detailed work for him, take over for him when he has to talk, yet not rob him of the prestige and glory that he feels is coming to him. His rationalization here follows: "I surely can do the work much better than most people. My only obstacle is that I stutter when I have to express myself. Therefore, since I was born to stutter, and can't help myself, I'm entitled to at least the praise and glory for my hidden talent and abilities. Others should recognize the 'truth'—that if I didn't stutter, how simply I would be able to master many of these same situations."

In job situations, however, he blinds himself to the reality that he avoids not only situations where he may have to speak, but many others. When this is brought to his attention, he may be forced to agree to this fact, but then quickly turns about and feels that situations in which he must talk do not enter into the picture and are of minor importance. He now feels that since he is so capable and intelligent he should not be made to work in inferior capacities. To a person of this sort, who places such a tremendous emphasis on the importance of speaking, any accomplishment of a different nature becomes degrading and worthless. He continues to shirk responsibilities and avoids competitive struggles, yet basically gripes and complains that he never gets a break in any field of endeavor. He narrows his activities and duties to a minimum. He feels constantly ill-used and harbors the attitude that he is being exploited and always has to do the "dirty work."

When the stutterer speaks, though he may fill in gaps of his discussion with distortions and contradictions, he demands that others shall understand fully what he is trying to say. Others should not be exacting and look for minor flaws in his remarks. They should understand that he really does know what to say, but that his stuttering makes his thoughts and words appear jumbled and confused. At times he may feel quite suspicious of others' immediate agreement with him. He then feels that what he did say could not have been too praiseworthy if it was so easily understood by others.

The person who tends toward stuttering is generally adverse to any form of coercion, implicit or explicit. In relation to others, he feels he should not have to be held to rules or regulations, regardless of their validity. He usually rebels aginst such rules, becomes indignant, and feels them as an imposition upon his privacy. He should not have to be at work at a specific time, regulate his time to bus or train schedules, or be subjected to questioning or examination. In situations where he cannot rebel or avoid feeling coerced, he retaliates by unconsciously protesting with the use of his stuttering.

Because he stutters, he feels he can make a claim to exempt himself from situations that are threatening to his weakened structure. This claim for immunity pertains not only to speaking situations but also to natural laws, psychic or physical, such as factors of time, weather, illness, accidents, bad fortune, or even death. Exemption is the most secret claim he makes on life. Toward suffering his attitude may be one of denial. He demands that he should not be affected by trouble and discontent when they occur. At other times, feeling maltreated, he stoically demonstrates the many ways in which he is inflicted with pain. He feels that since he has suffered in the past with his stuttering, he should in the present and future be entitled to a life devoid of personal problems. When difficult situations do arise in his daily activities, he feels indignant, protests violently, blames it on ill fate, and feels entitled to be relieved without having to go through the laborious process of changing. Though many people who stutter make all sorts of claims about wanting to help themselves become cured, the author has actually found very few who feel they want to make the sacrifices necessary for a solution of their problems. Their claim to be able to change without the slightest effort and their overemphasis on magic are serious obstacles in the curative process.

Finally, regarding claims, the person who stutters makes excessive demands on and holds magical expectations toward women in general. Aside from his more obvious claims toward women for absolute devotion, understanding, admiration, and surrendering love, he adheres to the belief that a woman magically can (as his mother did in the past), appear out of a blue sky whenever he feels in need of her. She should take over for him when he is in difficulty, remedy the situation, yet disappear and take on a minor role at other times. She should understand how sensitive a person he is and mold her own feelings and beliefs to his way of life.

The stutterer, because of his exaggerated sense of anxiety, is in constant battle with himself and feels like a helpless victim under relentless pressure a great deal of the time. Even when he is not stuttering and is calm and relaxed, the slightest jar to his transient equanimity can set off and generate anticipatory anxiety. One patient has put it as follows: "I'm rid of pressure only when I'm sleeping or dead tired." This relentless pressure is rooted in part in the claim he makes, that it is "only fair and just" that in speaking situations he be given prior and sympathetic consideration. He feels coerced most times, under undue stress, and pushed mercilessly by the many imaginary demands on his environment. He does not experience these demands as resulting from his own entanglements; therefore, since others are to blame, he is then justified in demanding attention and consideration of others, and especially so in the speaking situation.

To such an extent and degree does the individual who stutters become a stickler for justice, justice for himself, that is, that it is a doubtful matter whether he would give up his stuttering if he could. He asserts his claims for prior and special attention and consideration in speaking situations by first feeling that his listeners are under obligation to bear with him. He then proceeds, via the tortured, fear-ridden route of his stuttering, to put his listeners through the wringer, testing them out, so to speak, with his repetitious speech, bodily contortions, blocks, arrhythmic gesticulations, sighs, and so forth.

The diffuse feelings of frustration and discontent experienced by the individual who stutters are in part due to anxiety related to speaking situations. This does not gainsay the fact that they are mainly due to disturbances in the overall character structure. The individual who stutters encapsulates all his frustrated feelings and his discontent into what he considers his speech handicap. Nevertheless, it is not the speech situation nor the speech difficulty as such, but his investment in it that determines the degree and frequency of his stuttering.

If he is moving against people, his aggressiveness is expressed in the explosive nature of his speech. If clinging, his stuttering can be the helpless whimperings of the child. If moving away from people, his justification and his excuse for his compulsive need to withdraw lies ready to hand—his stuttering. He doesn't want to stutter. People make him stutter; so he keeps away from people.

In treatment the stutterer feels that his mere presence in therapy is a claim to being cured. This claim is backed up by two rationalizations: (1) Because of his stuttering he has suffered a lot and been deprived of many things that would otherwise have come his way, and (2) he has read extensively about the problem of stuttering. In short, his suffering because of his stuttering has purified him and made him in character a better person than others. His extensive reading and wide knowledge about stuttering endow him with added strength, for knowledge is power.

On the other hand, he tends to feel abused when it is pointed out to him that to help himself he had to make extensive efforts and sacrifices in areas of his personality and overall character structure that may seem to have little direct bearing on stuttering or not stuttering. He feels he should be able to help himself solely on the premise of his intellectual awareness and the suffering that he has had to endure as a stutterer.

He feels that he should be able to "conquer" his stuttering by sheer conscious control. He should be omnipotent enough to "master it" with the slightest of effort. Operating in this context is another *should* that remains largely unconscious. This should demands of him that he should be able to turn on his stuttering when it suits him and turn it off when it doesn't. For example, when he feels helpless and a need to cling, he should be able to (and does) exploit his stuttering for all it's worth and without compunction. But when he wants to shine, to command, and to convince, he should be able to by calling on his willpower to speak fluently and impressively and to not stutter at all.

Any failure in this direction is met on his part with irritability, anger, rage, causing him to generate further anxiety and reactivate the stuttering. Many a person who stutters has found himself repeating, "This next time I must not and will not stutter. I must have the willpower to control it at all costs." Repeated failures do not cause such a person to take stock of himself honestly but drive him further into imposing impossible shoulds upon himself. His demands upon himself become coercive in nature and cause him to feel torn and ever more and more conflicted precisely because of the contradictory nature of these same shoulds. The result is a vicious circle that develops and spirals and keeps the individual in a constant state of conflict and unhappiness.

When these conflicts rooted in his own shoulds become unbearable, the person who stutters may then resort to externalization. That is, he may impose his shoulds upon others and feel that others should always be just as perfect. When others do not approximate perfection he then feels embittered and angered. An example of this may be implied in the rationalization that because he stutters and does not speak "perfectly," then he can and is entitled to demand perfection of others in the speaking situation. He may experience these expectations of himself primarily as coming from the outside and be quick to blame others for his own shortcomings. He may now feel that others cause him to stutter or others expect too much of him when he speaks; he, therefore, becomes rattled and unnerved and stutters. He may feel, as he does many times in speaking, that he is being coerced into saying exactly what others expect from him. As a result he feels pushed and inwardly pressured to the extent that he quickly becomes anxious. The stuttering that follows is compulsive.

He fails to understand here that these are his own inner demands and expectations in always wanting to be able to anticipate and measure up to everyone else's desire so that he can avoid being condemned, embarrassed, and criticized. To avoid feelings of hurt and rejection, he becomes extremely vulnerable and hypersensitive to any form of coercion, even if it is the most simple request. In this last sense the person who stutters is known for his sensitivity and rebelliousness to anything that he feels as being imposed upon him from the outside. He tends to become less and less rational and flexible and more and more stubborn and intractable.

In the speaking situation we do not see the actual outward manifestations of anger and rage. These feelings are held in check. What presents itself in their place is a facade of calmness and control. Beneath the facade, the individual feels coerced and forced to meet what he experiences as expectations coming from others. Anxiety and hostility begin to arise. The calm front is ripped apart as soon as he starts to speak. The stuttering that inevitably follows is an expression of rebellion.

What the individual who stutters fails to see at these times are his inner shoulds and expectations. He fails to see that *he is really his worst enemy*. Nevertheless there is an immediate gain for him, though a neurotic one. By externalizing the conflict to the outside and onto others, he can and does avoid the painful realization of his own shortcomings.

As a result of his constant shoulds, a feeling of strain is generated in him that has no letup. He suffers from a chronic state of exhaustion. He feels constantly on edge, tense, cramped, and hemmed in. He also feels to some extent a general restlessness. He feels depressed and in need of a great deal of sleep. His general musculature is tense, and there are feelings of rigidity and bodily contractures. The person who stutters feels in these periods all the more anxious and may tend to avoid most speaking situations. He begins to feel resigned, and his resignation may manifest itself into a tendency to withdraw from people and most activities and obligations.

As these inner dictates and shoulds, because of their impossible achievement, begin to fail, the neurotic superstructure begins to crumble. Self-hate enters into the picture. The baleful consequences of neuroses become more and more manifest.

The self-hate remains unconscious. The consequences of self-hate are felt more and more as frustration, dissatisfaction, diffused irritability, and so forth. In people who tend to stutter, these feelings themselves are related to failure in a speech situation, further obscuring the issue. Needless to say, the great base of the destructive iceberg remains submerged in the unconscious and covers many, many more areas of the total personality and is little related to failure in the speaking situation as such.

The tearing down of the superstructure, its crumbling, its rebuilding, and its reshaping, is a continual, dynamic, turbulent, and unceasing process. Internal pressures in the form of the shoulds and external pressures in the form of the claims fashion and embellish the neurotic superstructure. The very same shoulds and claims crumble and demolish it.

In the individual who stutters, his emotional complex is being exposed and tested every single moment of his life. And to be tested means precisely and concisely to fail. Failure then results in sensitivities and fears. He begins to avoid testing situations. He avoids those people who may demolish this neurotic superstructure of his. Moving inward, he narcotizes those feelings in himself that may endanger this superstructure. He creates numerous inhibitions so he may avoid this and that person, evade this and that issue. Even to himself he becomes slippery and illusive. "I can't understand what made me do it." is the alibi password perched like a crow on his lips picking at the putrefying corpse of his many failures to live up to his neurotic pride and to actualize his image.

As the superstructure of the individual who stutters continues to crumble despite his frantic efforts at rebuilding it and as the very foundations of his personality are shaken, he begins to hate himself more and more. But even here his hate is for his stuttering. He hates and despises himself as a stutterer. He hates himself for not being able to control his stuttering and "magic it away" when it is to his interest to do this. Nevertheless, behind this hate for his actual everyday self as a stutterer and growing out of it and reinforcing it is his hate for his real self. A startling idea festers in him. If it weren't for his real self holding him back and keeping him down, he could be a modern Demosthenes. But if it weren't for his real self he would be dead. He makes some desperate and sporadic attempts to restore balance, but finds himself further conflicted and divided.

The question is valid: If we can help the individual who stutters to reduce the extent and degree of his stuttering, would he hate himself less? The answer of course is yes. On the other side of the coin we encounter this question: Can the individual lessen his stuttering without first lessening the pressure of his shoulds and his claims? The answer is no.

Most of all we have seen that this emphasis on his stuttering as the cause of all his ills blinds the individual who stutters to his own self-hate. Furthermore, this blind emphasis on stuttering to the exclusion of other aspects of his behavior and his overall character structure adds to and reinforces his self-hate. Self-hate in turn feeds the pride from which it sprang in the first place. He seems caught in a dilemma. He hates himself because he stutters. His hate for himself reactivates the stuttering and compels him to stutter. His stuttering increases his hate for himself, and his hate for himself makes it extremely difficult for him to stop stuttering.

The consequences of self-hate in stuttering are varied and of a destructive nature. The first is in the compulsive need for people who stutter to constantly compare themselves with practically everyone with whom they come into contact. They place themselves at a disadvantage by feeling that the other person is usually the better speaker, more intelligent, better-looking, more interesting, more influential, etc. These comparisons are predominantly so in the speaking situation. The person who stutters unconsciously or consciously is constantly comparing himself to those about him when it comes to speaking. What he fails to see is that in his comparisons he really does himself an injustice. This latter comes about when he painfully chooses people with a superior talking ability with whom to compare himself. For example, he will destructively choose to compare himself with experienced and eloquent speakers. As he sits there quietly listening, he beats himself and becomes filled with anxiety and apprehension when he discovers that he himself is nowhere near this stage of development. He will belittle himself and undergo a self-destructive berating for not being able to approximate other speakers. In relation to those people with whom he is in closest proximity, he will also disparage himself by feeling that the others are more intelligent, wittier, glib, and possessed of more shining qualities generally. The person who stutters in these instances may feel inferior and in this process of self-criticism will slowly withdraw himself from others, increasing all the more his obsession of himself as a victim of society. As a result of all this, he becomes further resigned and hopeless and indirectly adds to the process of self-hate.

The person who stutters will find that as a consequence of self-hate, he will often take too much abuse from others. Because of his tendency to bend over backward at times and as a result of his compulsively compliant nature, he finds himself of necessity to be easily exploited and abused. Such an individual also feels that he is different from others, inferior to most people, and therefore may develop the idea that in reality he deserves little more.

A last consequence of self-hate is the need to balance it with the attention, regard, appreciation, admiration, or love of others. This striving for blind acceptance proves to be a very painful and compulsive pursuit, especially so in people who stutter. This is so because he fears standing alone and constantly throws himself and becomes totally dependent on others for self-evaluation. In the speaking situation, although he may experience himself as standing alone on the platform, he is also totally subjugated and dependent upon his audience for his own self-existence. At these times, his whole structure may fall or rise with the attitudes of others toward him. This is true not only while he is speaking, but before he begins to speak and after he has finished, when he may find himself frantically clutching at others and seeking the audience's reaction to his perfect "performance." At this time he feels as though he were thrown to the lions and is entirely at the mercy of others.

As these consequences increase in intensity, so does the person who stutters feel all the more imprisoned in his conflicts. His self-hate slowly mounts, and he finds himself in a vicious circle between pride and self-contempt. He is in the constant dilemma between becoming in his imagination the perfect orator or succumbing to the terror of being a horrible stutterer. One reinforces the other and, depending upon the situation, assumes greater or lesser propensity. This can change only to the extent that he becomes more aware of himself as a human being and can place his feet more squarely on the ground. It is then that he will be able to strive less toward imaginative heights and realistically look at himself as a person with a speech impediment, yet having many other human qualities, potentialities, and capacities that can be used successfully to lead a more or less healthy existence.

As the battle between pride and self-contempt becomes intensified, the person who stutters begins to become further frustrated and finds no relief from the strong persistent underlying sufferings that he undergoes. He is finally led to withdraw from others and to check his feelings, which become muted and unreal. He may then develop alternate feelings of uniqueness, turn to intellectualizations, and slowly undergo an inner withdrawal from himself in order to escape fully the pangs of this painful inner struggle. In withdrawing from others he slowly puts himself in a vacuum-like existence and may deaden his feelings all the more. The result of all this is that alienation from self slowly creeps in and eats at the core of his personality. Whatever realistic goals he may have to begin with, as a human being, become undermined and ignored; the person then continues to feel more empty, and as he maintains a thread-like existence with the world around him, he lives on the periphery of his personality and becomes barely involved with it. He may go on with the lifeless motions of a marionette or an automaton. He will exist in a vegetative state and not involve himself in any serious life endeavors. As he becomes more hopeless and develops an inner futility, he also hates himself and lives with the strong begrudging envy of one who sees life slipping through his fingers, being unable to do anything about it. Every aspect of life, be it social, educational, vocational, or personal, is affected. The handicap reaches into the lives of its victims and leaves a trail of suffering, sorrow, waste, and destruction.

Only through a change in the total character structure can self-hate lessen. As conflicting tendencies become lessened and the individual becomes less alienated and feels more of himself, he will then be able to feel less contemptuous of himself. At this time he will regard himself more as a human being, may become less involved in his stuttering as a crippling symptom, and will tend to use most of his energies toward living and self-realization and not toward self-destruction.

Chapter 4

ALIENATION IN STUTTERING

THE person who stutters, as a result of his faulty emotional makeup, has little feeling for himself. He feels remote and appears as a stranger to himself. He feels most of the time as though he were living in a fog. He does not feel himself as a human being with his own feelings, wishes, thoughts, and desires. He is robbed of most spontaneity; he has little or no initiative. In place of any real and alive feelings, he is a harried slave to compulsive and relentless drives.

In the process of stuttering, the individual finds himself divided within himself. He is possessed by many conflicting tendencies that rob him of experiencing himself as a whole. He has little feeling of his own body. He may appear to be hazy and confused, and his body sensations may be numbed. In the speaking situation, his own voice may be alien to him. When he speaks, he does not feel and experience his own voice as coming from himself and being his, but as coming from somewhere outside. Before he starts to speak, a glazed expression covers his face. He finds it extremely difficult to answer questions and comments or remarks addressed to him. He looks through people, rather than at them; a kind of mental paralysis and terror sets in at the mere idea of speaking before a group. He does not feel as though he is actually doing the speaking, but that of the speaking situation as being the more compelling and active force. He does not feel as though "I shall speak, I am speaking, or I will speak," but in terms of "I should speak, I must speak, and I have to speak."

Let us now try to see what may be the factors responsible for alienation from self. Firstly, the alienated individual is compulsively driven and feels very little of his own self as a moving force. For example, the person who stutters is not identified with himself at all, but rather with his poor image of himself. His feelings, thoughts, and actions, just as much as his voice and his speech, are estranged from him and alien to him. Before even beginning to speak, though he has spoken many times before in his life, and spoken well, he becomes highly anxious and apprehensive. He fears imaginary threats from his environment. He gets himself ready to ward off the attack. What he fails to see at these times is that the attack is actually coming from within himself. He likewise fails to see that what is being attacked is not himself, but his neurotic pride. He feels confused, becomes befogged, and can't think clearly. He is in constant threat that he won't be able to open his mouth the next time, that his voice will fail him, though actually he has spoken many times under the same circumstances.

The person who stutters depends mainly upon the spoken word for communication and self-expression. His exaggerated sense of responsibility for speaking robs him of spontaneity, flexibility, and a feeling for inner choice when expressing himself. Some stutterers are known to assume certain roles when speaking and to change to others at different times with little feeling or awareness. For instance, we know of those who can speak well in their capacities as teachers or administrator, yet stutter badly in other speaking situations. A change in social status can throw a stutterer's equilibrium off balance and cause him to feel threatened and chaotic. He may have little difficulty, for example, when talking to an inferior, someone he feels to have control over or toward someone who has to come to him for a favor, help, or information. His sense of "top and bottom," relationships, and position effect is a common indicator of the degree of alienation in stuttering. A sudden change in his social position causes him to feel tilted and confused, leading to anxiety and stuttering.

The stutterer is compelled to mold himself into something which he is not. He is pushed by a multitude of shoulds and musts, which are many times in complete opposition to what he really is all about. He strives to become in reality what he is in his imagination. He makes impossible claims upon himself, and his spontaneous energies as a result become hampered. He experiences himself as having special and endowed privileges. In place of his making his own decisions, he feels and demands that others take over for him. The person who stutters in this regard feels that since he is a stutterer, other people should make allowances for him. Because he is alienated from himself to some degree, he is not able to feel that his stuttering is his own problem and that it actually deters from his real self. Instead, he unconsciously makes himself into a cripple, increases his claims and demands upon the world, and actually increases his own conflicts, miseries, and sufferings.

Finally, there are the active moves against the real self as expressed in self-hate and self-contempt. In this respect the individual who stutters finds every speaking situation a new, bewildering, and confusing experience. He feels badgered and puts himself at the mercy of a magic broken record on the turntable in his mind that is stuck on the same timeworn tune, "This time I'm not going to stutter; I'll get by this time." He pushes the needle to the place where the record woefully wails, "Did I cover it up? Did anyone notice it?" In place of trying to accept himself with his stuttering at these times, he instead baits himself all the more mercilessly and then drives himself into further blind alleys. Because of his degree of alienation, the idea of evaluating himself as he is, with his conflicts and his stuttering, becomes loathsome and terrifying. The terror becomes prominent when he is confronted with the discrepancy between what he feels he should be in his imagination, that is a flawless speaker, and what he actually is in reality, that is an individual with a speech difficulty. The person who stutters as he increases his self-hate becomes alienated from himself further by resorting to various maneuvers, magical rituals, and distractions to cover up his own stuttering. He develops numerous devices and tricks to avoid the *bugaboo* word. The very ritual of stuttering seems an alienated process in itself. He also brings into play at the same time an arsenal of defensive protective measures, in order to allay and avoid any further anxiety. As a result he finds himself even more entangled, more confused, and anxious, his speech difficulty is increased, and he thus becomes all the more alienated from himself.

When he is through speaking, he finds himself lost, shaking, and fumbling blindly to return to his previous resigned state. His environment now appears even more strange and new to him. People who were just objects while he spoke and struggled with his stuttering become people once again. As he tries to get hold of himself, his immediate response is usually one of "What have I said? Was it clear? Were they able to understand me?"

He needs constant reassurance and reaffirmation from others. With monotonous repetitiveness he asks, "How was I? Did I have much trouble speaking? Did I stutter?" At the same time he fears and resents any reference to his stuttering and detests any kind of criticism, no matter how constructive it may be. He cares little whether he has contributed anything and whether he was interesting or stimulating. His speech, to the exclusion of everything else, is his greatest concern and worry. His egocentricity causes him to resort to the same persistent questions: "How perfectly did I speak? Were others impressed? Did I stutter?"

As a result of these moves away from the real self, there is a simultaneous alienation from self. In the individual who stutters this alienation is manifested in an inability to remember names, faces, and places. He feels himself impersonal and not belonging to himself. He shows a poor sense of direction. When caught unaware, he has great difficulty in giving his own name, age, and address. He rarely feels that what he says or feels as coming from within himself. He may feel that he is just one big bluff and lives in constant dread of being exposed. He hardly, if ever, stands on his own feelings or convictions. He is quick to fall back on the old bywords "so-and-so said it; it must be so; I read it in the newspapers; they say." He hides behind a cloak of authority and fears assuming responsibility or taking a stand himself. This adds to and increases further alienation and loss of his own real identity.

As a result of alienation from self, there are many effects on his personality and on his life as a whole. To begin with, his real and genuine feelings become hampered, inhibited, or diminished. He lives no longer in terms of his own feeelings, wishes, desires, or convictions, but is now governed by his pride. In the individual who stutters, the striving for glory is present mainly in the speaking situation. It is in this position that he feels himself more and more compelled to actualize his image of himself as the perfect speaker. Where the average speaker considers and gives due emphasis to what he has to say, the person who stutters is interested mainly in making a brilliant impression; he feels himself as being omnipotent and believes he must control his audience at all costs. His speech becomes uppermost. To him it is not what he is saying, but rather, how well is he speaking? He is not concerned about others, but is he stuttering this time or not? Because he is alienated from himself at these times, he does not experience his audience as being friendly, but feels they are there to criticize and to attack him at the slightest provocation, at any weakness that he may display. It is no wonder then that he feels afraid, threatened, and defensive and has to contend not only with his speech difficulty but also with his imagined critics. In those speaking situations where he feels the most threatened, he will experience his alienation to such a degree that he neither hears nor listens to himself when he is speaking. Oftentimes he may not even be able to identify with his own body, far less hear himself speak. He may feel threatened at the sound of his own voice. The very words he utters become both strange and dangerous to himself. What he has to say loses all meaning and significance even for him. He feels trapped and cornered and then the race begins: Hurry! Get it over with! Let the beginning be the end! Finish before the stuttering gets too bad! When he is through speaking, he feels frustrated, defeated, and hopelessly beaten. He is torn between remaining in the situation and returning to his audience for some understanding or sympathy, yet his pride interferes, for experiences of this sort he feels as being humiliating and embarrassing. He wants to return and magically straighten out what he believes had previously happened when he spoke, but when he cannot realistically do so, he then finds himself in further conflict. Should he remain and place himself at the mercy of his audience, or should he run and lose face? Both of these extremes are unbearable and offer no solution. One of his only resorts then is to alienate himself further from himself in order to numb his feelings and to remove himself from the actual situation. As one patient of mine described it quite well, "When I'm stuttering too badly, I begin to feel as though I am floating in thin air." Another time it is like "being up in the clouds. I then feel numb and I don't have to worry about what I said, or what others may be thinking about me at the time."

The individual who stutters lives with unresolved conflicts. As a result, there is a devastating waste of energies that are demanded not only by the existing conflicts themselves, but also by the all-around attempts to remove these conflicts. The individual who stutters, for instance, is forever worrying about his stuttering. A great deal of his energies go into these worryings over his stuttering. He also uses up a great deal of his energies in the conflicting and contradictory tendencies that are constantly being experienced by him. In the speaking situation, there is also a tremendous amount of energies that are being used up and misdirected in the overwhelming anxieties and apprehensions that are associated with the actual speaking. As more and more conflict becomes expressed in the foreground, more energy is taken away from the real self and becomes channelized in the area of self-idealization. Finally, the individual is left to feel inert, resigned, and hopeless about himself.

Much energy is also used up in the tremendous wavering and proscrastinating, which the individual who stutters is constantly involved with. Because of his inability to stand on his own feet and to take responsibility for his own actions, he finds himself in a constant state of indecision. He fears even taking responsibility for his own speech. As a result of all this, he cannot feel himself in the speaking situation. He is constantly plagued with thoughts and doubts as to when to talk. Should he leave it till later, will he stutter, etc.? He is in constant struggle with himself and with the world about him. With his constant maneuvering, evasions, and tricks, he is unable to feel any honesty about his own life. He keeps constantly externalizing his shortcomings and his speech difficulty onto others, refuses to bear the consequences of his own actions or decisions, and tries constantly to get by in any situation of responsibility. The mere fact that he refuses to accept responsibility by placing the blame on others for his stuttering further increases his problems. Finally, as the person who stutters becomes alienated, he loses even more of his integrating power, which is already at a low ebb. His ability to make decisions, to assume responsibility, and to have any spontaneous feelings can come about only from a resolving of his conflicts and a movement toward healthy self-realization.

The person who stutters does have cause for concern. He pays too great a price for the glory that he strives to achieve in his imagination. To travel that road can only mean alienation from himself and deadening and paralyzing inertia. He loses all zest for living and feels himself imprisoned and hopelessly resigned to a life as a stutterer. However, there is another road—that one leading to healthy growth and enjoyment of living.

As a consequence of stuttering, we find people who tend to hesitate in the speaking situation are chronic blockers in most other aspects of living. Since stuttering is a by-product of conflict, the stutterer ultimately incurs a paralysis of psychic energies, which affects not only individual initiative and action but also thought and emotion.

Rendered inert as the result of his unresolved conflicts, the person who stutters can rarely direct himself toward a goal. His center of gravity depends upon basic forces coming from outside himself rather than from within. When others do not meet his sensitive and impossible demands, he becomes frustrated and disoriented. The mere idea of extra effort on his part causes him to feel tired, unhappy, and even more justified in claiming for himself the special privileges that he regards as his natural rights.

Living with unresolved conflicts involves a devastating waste of energies expended not only on the conflicts themselves but also on all the roundabout attempts to remove these conflicts. An individual who is torn by conflict can never utilize all his energies constructively nor direct them toward any one whole-hearted purpose. Instead, he is always compelled to pursue two or more mutually incompatible goals. Such pursuit leads either to a scattering of energies or to a localized frustration. Ibsen's Peer Gynt perfectly illustrates the scattered energies in a person who is lured into the belief that he can achieve perfection in any endeavor. Such a compulsive need for superiority is often found in a man driven toward a controlling power in business, preeminence in the arts, and spectacular virtuosity in sexual activity. His feminine counterpart may strive simultaneously to be the ideal wife, the perfect hostess, the picture of fashion, and a practicing expert in extramarital affairs. Such an individual, no matter how gifted and versatile, inevitably succumbs disastrously to her own excessive demands. In the same way, the person who stutters drives himself relentlessly to create an image of "god-like" quality with which he can become not only "the great talker" but also "the gifted writer," "the epitome of humility and friendliness," and "a charmer and seducer of the masses." Such a person will ultimately find himself entangled in a web of conflicting tendencies.

The second and more common result of conflict living is the frustration of a single pursuit caused by the clash between incompatible motivations or drives. An individual may want to make friends but will be prevented from doing so by his domineering and demanding attitudes, of which he may be unaware. The stutterer, for example, feels constantly thwarted in the speaking situation because, although he may want to be gregarious, his stubbornness and need to be in control at all times defeats his purpose. In similar fashion, he may have a valuable contribution to make to a group but will want to present it in such a way as will glorify himself, for he is compulsively driven also toward being liked, respected, and admired and toward avoiding criticism and antagonism. Because of his need to excel and be outstanding, however, he externalizes his self-contempt and anticipates ridicule. All these efforts result in confusion and anxiety, with thought and action blocked, and the pertinent thought he might have contributed is lost by the wayside.

The person who stutters is a chronic hesitator in most areas of his life. His stuttering with all of its blocks and hesitations represents a more localized and externalized expression of his general state of indecisiveness and wavering. Before attempting to speak, he procrastinates and anxiously ponders over what to say, how to say it, and to say it at the most propitious time. He cannot be spontaneous in the choice of his words, and since speech is a conscious act to him, he is extremely cautious and perfectionistic in what he communicates to others. Even when he may feel quite certain about what he may want to say, his own self-doubts grow, and he then reverts back to a position of indecisiveness and further hesitation. In the end he finds himself in the dilemma of either offering passive resistance and refusing to say anything at all or involving himself further by pushing himself into making himself talk. Or, he may externalize the latter and feel that others are coercing him into speaking. As a result of all these conflicting tendencies, he becomes more entangled and rebellious, feels compelled and trapped, and grows more anxious and hostile—all of which finally leads to a state of confusion and stuttering speech. The tremendous expenditure of energy in a conflicting ordeal of this sort is bound to leave him frustrated, hopelessly resigned, inert, and exhausted.

MAGIC IN STUTTERING

In the period of early development, the child begins to recognize the importance of the effect of his parents and especially that of his mother upon its early development. This latter parent, the mother, begins to be experienced as a magic helper. Should this feeling of magic dependence be encouraged and promoted, then we may usually find the destructive sort of morbid dependency that characterizes mother-child relationships of overprotective, oversolicitous parents. The mother-child relationship is generally present in children who stutter. A child in such a milieu is rendered weak and insecure. As long as he can hide behind the cloak of his mother's authoritarian protectiveness, he may feel omnipotent and falsely secure. Should she, however, fail him at other times, he will then resort to all sorts of magic gestures in the manner of threatening maneuvers, such as whining and screaming, which are usually successful in this same relationship. He learns early in life the mastery and omnipotence of his magic gestures and uses these effectively until the day when reality in itself proves to him otherwise.

As the individual continues to grow and develop, he discovers even further the omnipotence of words and thoughts. With words he finds he can control and master things about him. Using the "right" or the "wrong" word can be of significant importance. "Words can kill and resurrect." "Words are dangerous, powerful, and destructive" and should be used with discretion. In people who learn to place an overemphasis on the omnipotent value in words early in life, such as may be found in those who develop stuttering, words become experienced as dangerous weapons. Words become filled with feeling and emotion. They can reveal one's innermost thoughts, feelings, hostility, or vindictiveness. Words can expose our most impenetrable defenses and readily reveal our truest personality.

From early development, especially in those individuals who tend toward stuttering, the spoken word carries with it an effect of tremendous imprint and impact. The child who stutters, for instance, learns early in life that speaking can upset his personality equilibrium and bring about inner chaos and the eruption of fear and anxiety. He also learns through experience that a mastery and control over his words is one of his only means of salvation. He finds it imperative to measure his words and to use them with utter care and caution, for "a careless word can cause a calamity." The speaking situation, to repeat, becomes his arena of combat— the one place where he can emerge the victor or succumb to the mercy of others. With a few words he should be able to convey the most difficult or comprehensive idea or thought, and magically his audience should immediately grasp its meaning and understand him completely. Because of the heightened magic and omnipotent significance placed upon speech by people who stutter, the urge to talk and its relationship to words becomes not only exaggeraged, but compulsive and indiscriminate in nature. Because of his inner hostility toward the world around him, he imaginatively attempts to triumph over others and to restore his hurt pride. To accomplish this, he attempts to cover up his frustrations by resorting to magic and to imaginative daydreams. Secretly, he wishes to occupy the center of the stage and to be the leader, the orator, etc. However, he adds to his sufferings and miseries by attempting to achieve these same heights through implied claims rather than through consistent efforts.

The person who stutters attempts to use most of his magic in the speaking situation, which is his greatest area of conflict. Since it is in this situation where he feels most threatened, concomitantly the greater the need for defensive measures and the use of magical solutions. In those most difficult speaking situations, such a person finds himself compelled to all sorts of magic in order to avoid exposure and feelings of anxiety, yet at the same time maintains a facade of self-containment.

Before the person who stutters even begins to speak, he usually feels apprehensive and afraid of what may happen to him in the speaking situation. His imagination may practically go wild with all sorts of self-torturing and self-recriminating doubts as to his ability to speak. He feels certain his jaws will lock and his mouth will remain tight shut the moment he decides to begin talking. In this process of self-hate and self-doubting there is some use of magic (a way out of the realm of actuality) in the manner in which he inflicts suffering upon himself. He may feel his audience as harsh and critical and as if they were placing the evil eye upon him the minute he begins to speak. He further aggravates his suffering by feeling and thinking that someone or other is staring directly at him and because of the way they look at him, they make him stutter all the more. In retaliation and as a defensive maneuver, such a person may then feel the greater part of his hostility toward these imagined enemies of his and as a result defensively puts himself in battle with his external world. He may feel now that his only recompensation is to strike back in order to restore his hurt pride and weakened position. Since at these times he has little real resources of his own to compete healthily with others, he is thus driven to resort to neurotic weapons, of which magic is one of his most powerful.

The position in which the person who stutters places himself in relation to his listeners is of prime significance and carries with it implications of magic. Choosing beforehand the right, the more strategic, or the safest position is one of his face-saving devices. These positions vary from person to person, situation to situation, and from time to time. There are those people who feel they can speak effectively only if they are sitting, others if they are standing, walking, etc. In relation to spatial concomitants, there may be those who according to their needs feel compelled to speak only when in the front, middle, back, or side of the room. Implied in these strategic positions is, no doubt, the implication of being magically able to control the situation and the external conditions at the time of speaking.

Though these peculiarities exist in many people when confronted with difficulties in the speaking situation, they seem to play a more intensified role in people who stutter. Since speaking is conscious in these people and because of the disruptive forces present in them when attempting to speak, they have a greater need for supporting mechanisms. To place himself in a superior position when threatened in a particular speaking situation aids the person who stutters to break through some of his fears and apprehensions. It also gives him some feeling of support in the belief of being able to shift magically from position to position or to dissolve into "thin air" if necessary. Before starting to speak, such a person takes pride in moving in and in beginning to speak when he feels his audience least expects it. In this maneuver of his, he not only assumes the superior position in throwing his listeners off guard, but can avoid within himself the fear of having to begin to speak at a specific time and "when others make him." In other words, he speaks at his own convenience, when he feels like it, thus avoiding the fear of coercion and being tied down to the specific. He also prides himself in feeling that his audience is taken by surprise, thrown off balance. By the time they can restore their equilibrium, he will have spoken and squeezed himself through another difficult and precarious position. Like a magician, he may feel he should blot out the existence of his stuttering to others and somehow not even be seen until he has completed speaking.

Each time a person who stutters speaks, he imaginatively and magically builds around himself a platform. He does not experience himself usually as conversing or talking with others, but pictures himself from an exalted position, speaking down to others. It is the magic omnipotence from this heightened position that adds to his difficulties in the speaking situation. One patient of mine was summoned to appear in court as a witness. He was informed that his own particular information would be limited to a few words and have very little bearing on the final results of the actual hearing. However, the mere idea of having to be questioned directly and specifically, and especially from a sitting position above others, terrified him to the point of not being able to open his mouth at all when called upon to give his testimony. Interestingly enough, in this period of panic and in the dilemma of not being able to speak, he turned to the judge, who sat at an even higher level than himself and magically gesticulated with his hands the need for a pad and paper. The judge understood and sympa-

thetically extended to him these implements, with which my patient was able to carry on and save face to some degree. I have re-
counted this incident in some detail to emphasize the terror that
most people who stutter are confronted with in speaking situations where they feel threatened. Their position at these times
becomes even more chaotic and precarious when their magic solutions begin to fail them. Not being able to evaporate and disappear
magically once they feel caught in such difficult dilemmas, they
become panicky and desperately attempt to use means to restore
psychic unit. These too begin to fail realistically, and since they
cannot face or admit to their own shortcomings, they turn to
another magic face-saving device: throwing themselves at the mercy of others. They assume shrinking and apologetic attitudes and
hope to be spared by others of some of the humiliation and ridicule, which they externalize as coming from others. Situations
of this kind, however, add little real knowledge or understanding
to many of these same persons' understanding of themselves. They
feel only all the more hostile and victimized.

The process of stuttering in itself is a ritual filled with magic
gestures. Just before a person who stutters begins to talk, he may
secretly whisper to himself those bugaboo words which he may
fear most in the speaking situation, desperately hoping that such
a magic gesture will erase further difficulty. He feels that he
should be able to use sheer willpower and rigid conscious control
over his speech, in spite of having realistically stuttered many
times before. He may feel "nothing can happen to me this time;
I must never stutter again." As he attempts to speak, he omni-
potently lifts himself in imaginative stature, feels himself above
others, and attempts by magic to control his audience.

When speaking, the person who stutters feels threatened and
as a defense against anxiety that he can magically throw his
voice out to his audience or pull it back into himself. In covering
up his fears he plays with words, changes them about, substitutes
some for others, and may even go to the extent at times of creat-
ing his own vocabulary when in difficulty. Driven for emotional
survival, he feels he must be the master of his own language and
should magically use it to suit his own particular needs. It is by no
means unusual to hear him coin a word or express unfamiliar

sounds or gesticulate as he stutters. The stutterer may become annoyed, however, if you should not by some magic implications understand the meaning of his cryptic verbal communications. To the person who stutters with all of his claims on magic acceptance, bizarre feelings and experiences of this kind are not too rare. He may also feel at other times that by mental telepathy others should understand the message or idea he is trying to convey as he stutters. At still other difficult times when speaking, as a face-saving device he attempts to cover up his difficulties by filling in gaps with falsities, using absurd rationalizations, or even obvious distortions. If questioned at these times as to the validity of his remarks, he is taken aback with surprise and feels enraged at others for what he feels as being unfairly questioned and embarrassed. What he is really taken aback by is rage at himself for not having reinforced and made foolproof his magic solutions. Others should not see through his defenses, otherwise he is a poor magician, and others might think him a bluff and a phoney. Here again we see the extent of this blind belief of his and the compelling need in his magic maneuvers and duplicities. These irrational desires, however, fail him as he becomes further entangled in his own conflicting and contradictory actions.

In the more severe forms of stuttering, one can vividly witness the overt display of the use of magic in the bizarre and grotesque speech behavior patterns sometimes presented at the height of speech difficulty. For instance, the stutterer may begin by discussing a serious matter, suddenly have difficulty in speaking, and anxiously switch into a phase of many sorts of compulsive, indiscriminate, and disorganized movements. At the point of interruption or hesitation, when the state of anxiety and disruption is usually at its highest level of tension, such an individual may suddenly stop speaking, interrupt his trend of thought, then by magic suddenly begin to whistle, giggle, smile, splutter, or mumble or give vent to an explosion of words. Some may, at these periods of chaos, suddenly again break away from the original discussion, start to tell a joke, or even continue by telling something completely out of context with the original idea or premise. In this ritual of unconscious magic maneuvering, it is the hidden need of such a person to erase any indication of stuttering to his own awareness and especially from that of his listeners. This same person when in conflict magically attempts to keep those around him in a state of disorganization and confusion long enough to give him time enough to pull together his own chaotic state and move through the difficult period of stuttering with little injury to his hurt pride. Little does he know that his hesitations and other manifestations of stuttering might be less oblivious and painful to himself and others than his distorted magic rituals, which rarely function and which are quite obvious and easily exposed by others. In reality, he actually increases the precariousness of his weakened position in these manifestations of his by engendering additional attention toward his speech impediment.

The various bodily movements and contortions used by a person when he stutters also carry with them a sense of implied magic ritual. The pressing of both hands against the sides of the body, the pinching of himself to get started, the blinking of his eyelids, the placing of the palm of his hand over his mouth, etc., are just some of the many bodily magic gestures used in a particular difficult speaking situation. Each one, I'm sure, has a particular unconscious omnipotent and magic meaning to suit specific neurotic needs at the time of conflict. It would be too time-consuming to elaborate on each one of these individually or to enter into any detailed psychoanalytic explanation of their possible implied significances. At this point I feel it suffices to say that as a whole they are unconscious attempts to hold together magically what is felt as disruptive and chaotic at the time in their individual organisms. By magic, stutterers feel they should and must hold together their disorganized personalities, such as by pinching themselves into aliveness and spontaneity, covering up the flaws in their character armor, mastering their language and faculty of speech by playing with and changing their words to suit their own needs, and, finally, blotting out of their awareness and that of their listeners' any weakness or discrepancies in their "perfect" image of themselves. These attempts at magic fail many times and may appear to be utterly fantastic; yet in understanding the person who stutters, it is important to keep in mind the tremendous amount of neurotic pride invested in these same magic solutions. He dares not and cannot give them up and cannot lose faith in them and fears losing hold of them, for without them he experiences himself as being lost, nothing, deadened, and prey to the onslaught of his anxiously waiting self-hate. To give up these irrational attempts at solution can come about only through a slow unveiling and resolution of his conflicts as a whole.

There is also an air of magic to the reactions of the person who stutters soon after each speaking situation. He magically feels at these times that he should erase whatever stuttering or difficulty he may have just experienced previously. Though he may have just completed an episode of anxious and chaotic manifestations or seemingly obvious hesitation and stutter-like speech, he suddenly controls himself to assuming a facade of utter indifference and calmness. His fear of social disapproval compels him to assume the attitude of "What's all the excitement about? Nothing has really happened," or "You see, what you may have just witnessed was just an accident. I'm really a very poised and relaxed person." This attempt toward automatic rigid control seems to help such a person for the moment, but his own self-doubts and self-recriminations gnaw at his inner structure. Since he cannot stand to admit any flaws or discrepanices in his godlike makeup, he finds it necessary to deny these same things to himself and to others. And, finally, since he cannot stand his own evaluations, assertions, or convictions, he is relentlessly driven to turn toward others for their opinions and approval of himself.

Following a difficult speaking experience, though such a person knows to some degree the extent of his stuttering, he is still driven to turn to others for their opinions and evaluation of his performance. What he really hopes for here in a magic sense is not a realistic impression of his flaws, but the imaginative wish that others may not have noticed his stuttering. If such may be the case at times, he still feels anxious and threatened to the point of further self-doubt and self-recrimination. Instead of saving face and leaving things well alone, he may now turn to his listeners and say "How was I, by the way? Was anyone impressed by what I said? How did I look, how did I speak, was I poised, did I give a good delivery, was my enunciation clear enough, was my voice loud enough, was anyone bored as I spoke, etc." The latter may be somewhat exaggerated, but part or most of these questions are present, I feel sure, to some extent either in an implicit or explicit manner in the minds of most people who stutter.

As the person who stutters is compulsively driven to turn to his listeners for their approval, criticisms, and reaffirmation, so does he want to be able to maintain his superiority by pretending to be aloof from and independent of others. In this search of his for magic illusions, should he be confronted by others with the realities of his performance in the speaking situation, he feels further threats to his weakened structure and magically turns the table by repeating to himself an old face-saving device: "Sure, I've done badly this time, but the next time there will be no more stuttering." Or, in these periods where he has to repress his real feelings of hurt and disappointment when face to face with the realities in himself, he resorts to the device of completely numbing his feelings and assuming the appearance of utter poise and calm as though nothing had happened. In this forced psychic masquerading phase, he may suddenly drop the avid interest he had in interrogating others about himself and may change the scene from seriousness to one of comedy or flippancy. He can now suddenly wipe away his tears of frustration and become the clown or joker of the crowd. By such an elusive gesture calculated to regain superiority and to mend any perforations in his exposed and wounded pride, he attempts to regain the center of the stage. In this bitter position he deceives himself into believing that he can resign himself to "fate," that he can "laugh things off," and that his stuttering isn't too bad after all. He may be compelled to carry this cynicism even further by telling others about these futile feelings of his and joking or making fun of them. He may tell a few jokes about people who stutter, placing them in the most embarrassing and difficult positions he can imagine, and may even mimic them with his own stuttering. In this process of degrading himself, he feels that he can at least compensate for his previously weakened position by raising himself magically to a second and more omnipotent platform: being on stage as the "star of the show." Feeling trapped by his own maneuvers, he now believes in his own blind and alienated sense: "I must be twice as good to be able to regain the confidence of my audience from a defeated position." His pride in magic gains strength and momentum at these times, for it adds to his alienation in believing that "nothing can touch or hurt me. I'm too keen and quick. I can make others forget my flaws and admire me just the same." He also adds to his feelings of omnipotence in pretending to himself that like a magician of the theater he can imaginatively change, switch, or recreate scenes in order to get the maximum effect from his audience. Little does he comprehend that in these maneuvers of his and with his attitudes of indifference and superficiality, he is basically adding fuel to his already weakened personality structure.

Should he not be able to seduce or manipulate his audience with all his magic array, he may find himself in real danger. With his back to the wall, and feeling helplessly trapped in his own maneuvering schemes, he can resort only to one last weapon: externalization. He now approaches his listeners with annoyance or even rage and blames them for his difficulties and shortcomings in the speaking situation. At these times his blind belief in his own falsifications and dissensions may be so strong as actually to make him feel righteously justified. He may withdraw himself from others and boast of his decision to never to speak to these people again or have anything to do with them. In this forced withdrawal and retreat he magically attempts to save the day by distorting the actualities and externalizing his problems onto others, onto the outside. This play of mirrors is so deeply unconscious that even the stutterer is sometimes unaware of its operation.

The person who stutters frequently makes inexorable magic claims upon others. The more stringent of these claims is the obsession that a blind quest for love will serve as a comprehensive solution to all his problems. He may be compulsively driven to feel that by receiving love and understanding from others his conflicts will automatically disappear, leaving him a free and happy individual. At times this need for affection can become so great as to serve as one of life's motivating forces. His mistake is in confusing a neurotic need for affection with a real capacity for love. What the stutterer is actually searching for is magically to expect and demand from others "absolute devotion," "blind admiration," and "surrendering love."

The person or persons toward whom such magic claims are directed usually represent some position of superiority or strength according to the particular need of the stutterer and may be frequently changed as the need or situation changes. Such a person may be a parent or other relative, an employer, a sex partner, a marital partner, etc. The male stutterer usually turns to a woman as his symbol of magic helper. A woman is symbolic of what his mother once represented to him: "a magician at all times, ready in all emergencies, regardless of the nature of the situation."

In adulthood we may find these absolute claims upon women to be a part of a more complex and involved process. A stutterer will be attracted to a partner who may impress him as being stronger than and superior to others and who can serve as an unconscious protection against his own weakened and precarious situation. For he feels that if he can depend upon his own choice of partner for protection and safety, then he can become invulnerable to the many hurts and frustrations he experiences as coming from the hostile world around him.

The stutterer magically expects this partner to surrender herself totally to all his whims and needs as they arise. She should magically foresee any difficulties he may have, especially in the speaking situation. She should cover up for his stuttering and talk for him whenever she senses he might begin to stutter without exposing his impediment or embarrassing him in the presence of others. Not only should she be able to meet these emergencies at all times, but she should be able to do so with poise and grace without making him feel weakened or foolish. She should move magically in and out of his more difficult speaking spots without being too obvious about it, and should always be sufficiently keen and alert not to assume too much the center of the stage. She should then withdraw at an opportune moment, allowing him to reenter nonchalantly and resume his starring role with éclat and a semblance of strength.

Even though he may consider his partner the superior and stronger one, the stutterer secretly believes himself to be the master and real magician. Nevertheless, he expects perfection and godlike qualities in her, demanding that each time she be better than the last. In this claim of his, he externalizes onto his partner his own hidden omnipotent and power-driven motives. He imaginatively believes that he could attain heights of mastery and perfection if only his partner would give him the support, the protection, and the safety, which he feels is his rightful due.

His partner should magically turn on and off her emotions to suit his particular moods. She should guess, without his communicating to her, those moments in which he may feel lonely, saddened, hurt, or even conflicted. At these times he may demand from her all sorts of reactions, ranging from understanding, sympathy, closeness, and warmth to wanting to be left alone in utter privacy. At still other times there may be a complete switch of his own feelings to gladness, joy, elation, or even hilarity. He will expect her to feel similarly and react accordingly, no matter what her own personal feelings or reactions may be at the time.

I feel that the symptom and the greater part of the ritual of stuttering itself is a major attempt toward an unconscious magic gesture with the purpose of symbolically demonstrating to others how the person who stutters suffers and is victimized. The dual effect, of course, is to perpetuate the feelings of much deeper, buried resentment and hostility toward his external environment as a whole and at the same time to be able to strike out and express his own hidden aggressiveness without fearing too great a retaliatory effect in return. It also serves to protect and ward off any possible imagined fears of self-disintegration and self-destructiveness in the person himself. I feel strongly that the magic implicit in this unconscious mechanism, with all its invested pride and omnipotence, gives explanation and purpose to the tenacity of the symptom of stuttering in general. In this comprehensive solution of his, the person who stutters can magically strike back at his early imagined enemies, protect himself at the same time from inner or external retaliatory effects through his martyr-like assumed attitudes, and finally attempt to achieve perfection and god-like heights with his facade of humility and honesty.

The use of magic solutions in the problem of stuttering produces destructive and adverse consequences to the personality of these individuals as a whole. The use of magic by a stutterer represents the degree of alienation and the degree of self-idealization, with its imaginative qualities. To remove these attempts at magic in such people without first building some inner foundation of strength and confidence would only defeat its own purpose.

Chapter 5

THE SPEAKING SITUATION
IN STUTTERING

THE onset of verbal communication begins early in life. The child at this period of development discovers that he is able to express through words and gestures his inward wants and desires. He also discovers that he is not a totally independent being, but dependent upon his environment for acceptance and social approval. He further discovers that his earliest conflicts become expressed in his communications, both verbal and social, in relation to his parents. When serious conflicts arise, the protective structures of a child's organism become threatened, anxiety is generated, and it is in the specific area of verbal communication that it is first experienced and expressed. Finally the speaking situation, which is normally used to convey an opinion, an attitude, a feeling, or an assertion, becomes a situation identified and experienced with fear and hostility. The speaking situation automatically becomes a conscious act, and the forerunner of future difficulties and uncertainties in such a disturbed child. Each subsequent attempt to speak, when under similar conflict, is met with further increasing doubt, fear, apprehensions, and anxieties. The hesitation that results and crystallizes into what is later known as stuttering results from the conflict between a rational desire to speak and express one's self and the opposing conflicting situations that arise as a result of speaking.

As the stuttering process is formed and develops into a more integrated entity in the adult, so does the speaking situation add onto itself additional complexities. This is especially so in the person who stutters, where the speaking situation is of specific significance. Though each individual conveys his own specific attitudes and feelings in his own particular communication, certain types of prevailing attitudes or peculiarities may be distinguished among people who stutter in any particular speaking situation. These attitudes may be classified as: (1) attitudes toward himself, that is the speaker; (2) attitudes toward others, that is the auditors; and (3) attitudes toward the person or thing spoken about.

ATTITUDES TOWARD HIMSELF

The very intention to speak has an objectional significance to the person who stutters; the mere thought of speaking carries with it a common denominator of fear, dread, and apprehension. The person who stutters starts with the feeling that the speaking situation is a dangerous situation and one in which he is bound to fail. His organism is set immediately into gear for an imaginary battle, which he perceives as about to begin once he starts to talk. Inwardly he feels anxious, disorganized, confused; his physiological and emotional response is chaotic and disruptive. These diffuse and extreme reactions originate usually even before the utterance of a single word and are entirely out of proportion to the realities of the situation. Anticipatory reaction of fear and a dread of speaking may be present in any of us before speaking situations that threaten our particular personality structure, such as speaking before a group, appearing in court as a witness, etc. However, to the person who stutters, almost any intent to speak, be it threatening or not, is experienced with marked anxiety and with a diffuse feeling of fright. Since the stutterer has had repetitive experiences of difficulties in speaking since a child, for him the speaking situation continues to be experienced as an automatic threatening situation, no matter what the actualities of the experience itself.

Where this anticipatory dread in the average speaker varies in degree and intensity, it usually also lessens or disappears once he begins to speak. In the person who stutters, however, his entire organism is usually involved to the extent that he alienates and dissociates himself intermittently from the situation. His anxiety and fears usually culminate to a practically uncontrollable degree so that he feels compelled either to take flight from speaking altogether and thus avoid the unpleasantness of the situation or else enter into this same situation with a feeling of doom, confusion, and doubt as to its ultimate outcome. With such a pessimistic outlook before speaking, it is easy to understand how he will ultimately feel and present himself in the speaking situation itself.

Once the person who stutters finally decides to take the felt dreaded plunge into speaking, he still does not adapt himself to depend upon his own natural resources for spontaneous verbalization. He now feels that his one possibility in breaking through the dilemma of speaking is to resort to various learned maneuvers, evasions, substitutions, and magical rituals. He can substitute an easy word for a feared word, add extraneous words to help him over difficult spots, postpone the utterance of a sound by the use of *ah-ah*, or even change the entire context of what he is saying at the time to suit his own devices. Other ways of momentarily releasing anxiety in the speaking situation are distractions of all sorts, such as pinching himself, talking in a mechanical tone, laughing at a moment of anticipation, looking away, or drawing the listener's attention by some non-speech activity. These releasing devices aid the person who stutters to break through a hesitation or block in speaking, though they are basically artificial in nature and actually intensify and engender the stuttering itself in a speaking situation.

These first components of disturbance and behavior disorganization that occur in the person who stutters are basically of an emotional or feeling variety. They occur usually when such a person's organism is set into gear in response to an anticipatory dread resulting from stimuli relating to the speaking situation. The effect, as has been stated, is of such a chaotic and disruptive nature that there is a marked discrepancy between the response and the actuality of the situation. Finally, these affective responses are specific to the individual and occur with an automatic trigger effect, causing the particular person to stutter when in a particular threatening speaking situation.

The second stage in the stuttering process has to do with the many complexities involved in the thought processes preceding the actual verbalization of the spoken word. In this difficult preverbal formative period, the person who stutters must contend not only with the actual thought or the meaning of what he is to say, but many of his energies now become directed toward how he should say it, when he should say it, also to be able to say it without hesitation or difficulty. He must be able to speak clearly, perfectly, concisely, and flawlessly. He must also keep out of awareness stimuli that have caused him difficulty when having spoken in the past. He attempts the latter by keeping the various devices mentioned in smooth operation and under perfect control. Since all of these are in urgent need of attention and take energy away from any spontaneous verbalization, what results instead is usually confusion, hesitation, and blocking, both of thought and of language. The ultimate result is one of increasing difficulty in speaking, added anxiety, continued dread, further confusion, and blocking, thus setting into operation a vicious circle.

The average speaker usually experiences his speech as his own and as originating from within himself. He feels a choice of his own words or group of words, though there may be some indecision as to word pronunciation. Once he makes his decision and voluntarily chooses his words, he will have little difficulty in consummating the speaking itself. The person who tends to stutter, however, generally experiences his speech as alien to himself and as coming from somewhere outside of himself. As a result of his inner turmoil, he experiences little choice in deciding upon one or another word, but must choose between word entities. His dilemma in speaking is experienced not so much in terms of what to say but how to say it with all of its explicit and implicit perfectionistic claims.

The person who stutters colors a great deal of his speech with the particular mood or feelings he may be experiencing at the time he is speaking. He is unable to keep these varying reactions to himself, but feels compelled and driven to project his feelings when speaking into his particular speaking situation. Since the success or failure of what he says is highly dependent upon the acceptance or disapproval of others, he gears his speech to meet and suit what he feels as demands coming from others. This accounts for the many mood fluctuations that are characteristic of people who stutter and that may tend to explain the fact that such people are stutter-free in one particular situation but may stutter severely in another.

The intense emotional disruptions that occur in people who stutter result not from fear of speech, but from fear of the speaking situation. No two speaking situations are alike either in meaning or effect. Though the person who stutters fears most speaking situations, he has the greatest difficulty in those situations that represent the greatest threat to his particular basic structure. The more pride is invested in his idealization of becoming the perfect speaker the greater the fear in those particular speaking situations. In such people the speaking situation is not experienced as a situation where normal verbalization can be expressed. Instead, it becomes threatening, and the person who stutters, with all of his hypersensitivities, is driven to feel in a state of constant apprehension and anxiety while in the situation. As a result of his diffuse and disturbing feelings, his speech becomes inhibited and blocked in many ways. What could be a natural and ordinary way of talking now becomes the hesitating and repetitive speech, which we know as stuttering. Similarly, speaking situations at one time or another in the past have become so conditioned that similar situations are experienced beforehand as situations of danger. Although the conditions of a particular speaking situation may occur under entirely new circumstances, the remembrance of past difficulties in speaking set up a trigger factor for a possible repetition of the stuttering in this same situation. The person who stutters because of his conflicting tendencies is usually unable to evaluate the realistic conditions in a situation. His responses to a speaking situation are governed mainly by compulsive and indiscriminate drives that come from his image of himself and not from his real self.

As the person who stutters loses more of his real identity, his role in the actual speaking situations becomes of a more alien and artificial nature. He anticipates each subsequent speaking occurrence as a fearful situation, with increasing doubts and hypersensitivities. With each new onslaught of anxiety and dread associated with the thought of speaking, his basic confidence becomes weakened. His only recourse now, he feels, is to either escape and avoid the situation or to gear himself for combat. In either case he is prone to self-recriminations, self-criticisms, and varying affective responses of an anxiety nature. Should he attempt to dare to speak, he feels little conviction of succeeding in the specific speaking situation, but instead enters into it with a feeling of either failure or hoping to squeeze through or get away without stuttering. Speech, which is usually involuntary, becomes a conscious act to him, and as he becomes more anxious and afraid, the more he entangles himself, leading ultimately to hesitation and blocks in his speech.

In any particular speaking situation, the average speaker does have some degree of control over the situation and can decide upon a course of action without too much emotional imbalance. The stutterer, who is fearful and anxious when he must speak, is usually unable to help himself predetermine his behavior before speaking. He may attempt to alleviate dread and uncertainties by communicating with himself the thought that he will not become frightened or that he will speak slowly and easily or avoid the feared words. However, when the actual time for action occurs, his hypersensitive organism to stress seems to return to its previously disruptive and chaotic state.

Another blocking stone to the person who stutters is his rigidity to change, his incapacity to become flexible in the speaking situation itself. The average speaker will voluntarily stop speech when he anticipates or is in difficult speaking circumstances. He is able to interrupt his speech when he may feel some disturbance and to resume his speaking at a more suitable level of productivity. The person who stutters, however, tends to sabotage his own self-interests when in a speech difficulty and activates the unpleasantness of his unfavorable position. The slightest indication of blocking or hesitation before or during the process of speaking disrupts his organism to an even greater degree of imbalance and chaos. For to have to admit discrepancies or flaws to his own notion of perfection is a severe blow to his pride. Since he should not have any flaws in his speech, and especially since he should remain unruffled when he does demonstrate hesitations in talking, his protective structure becomes dented and is then experienced as irreparable. He now has to contend not only with an immediate magical restoration of his crumbling superstructure, but is also subject to all the recriminations, embarrassments, and criticisms, which he externalizes to the outside. At these times the person who stutters becomes overwhelmed with an attitude of disaster and with a feeling of too little strength or volition on his part of being able to do anything about his precarious position. In these chaotic states he feels completely and compulsively driven by forces outside himself, at the mercy of his stuttering. He can only desperately hope to salvage part of himself and magically wish for some restoration of himself, yet feat at the same time complete doom and disintegration.

With each repeated failure in the speaking situation, the person who stutters feels increasing frustration and defeat. He becomes further divided within himself and as a result is more alienated from himself. He is driven into additional repetitive vicious circles of dread, fear, anxiety, hesitation, and blocks, and finally the conflicts themselves become crystallized in the form of stuttering. With each subsequent reversal in the speaking situation, such a person feels all the more driven to believe that "the next time" he will speak with greater perfection. He justifies his abused feelings and tends to exaggerate his attitudes of being a victim of society. He develops more stringent shoulds or expectations upon himself, makes more demanding claims upon others, and compulsively drives himself in repetitive states of chaos and inner disruption. The final outcome of such a process are consequences of an adverse nature, leading finally to inertia, resignation, and hopelessness. His actions no longer become voluntary but dependent upon the necessities of the speaking situation as it presents itself.

The more inadequate and inferior the stutterer experiences himself to others, the more he has to prove himself in the next speaking situation. He feels compelled to compensate for his feelings of uncertainty and insecurity each time he thinks about or actually participates in the act of speaking. What he fails to see here is that what he is actually driven to prove is not his real position in the speaking situation, but that of his idealized image of himself as the perfect speaker. The speaking situation, to the person who stutters, represents a comprehensive neurotic solution in which he attempts to solve all his conflicting tendencies. His intentions may be good, but his solutions are unhealthy and can lead only to further stuttering.

ATTITUDES TOWARD OTHERS, I.E., THE AUDITOR

The person who stutters is strongly dependent upon the reactions of his audience, whether it is one or more people. What he fears in the speaking situation depends to some degree on how he may feel he performs in the act itself and to a large extent also upon the expectant response he anticipates from his listener. Toward others, when he speaks, he may experience himself as though he were on stage. He then sees himself as the performer at the mercy of his critics, the audience. The latter response varies as to the particular situation in itself, and the degree of anxiety or threats varies to the particular neurotic structure that are experienced at the time. The more threatening an audience appears, the more intensely he will fear the situation itself, and the greater the amount of criticism or rebuff will be experienced as forthcoming.

In relation to others, the person who stutters is in constant need of their approval, praise, recognition, and reassurance. He feels that since he stutters he can make claims upon others for their absolute understanding, sympathy, consideration, and attention. Since he feels at most times geared in battle with imaginary enemies, he externalizes these hostilities, and he feels at the mercy of others as a result. Because of his extreme sensitivity to coercion, criticism, rebuff, or the slightest denial, his audience looms up all the greater as a threat to his particular neurotic structure. The person who stutters not only has to contend with his own internal turmoil and with his efforts to speak correctly, but also must meet the imagined expectations he feels as coming from his audience. It is no wonder that such a person's organism is thrown into further chaos, and a vicious circle ensues.

The auditor's response to a stutterer is of utmost significance, and the listener can control to a large extent the stutterer's feeling responses in the speaking situation. From his speaking position the stutterer feels thrown completely on his own resources and feels utterly alone and unable to lean on anyone or anything. In this terrifying isolated state in such a threatening situation, he may then compulsively turn to his old maneuvers, evasions, or magical solutions, but at one time or another these all seem to fail him. The more such defenses begin to fail him, the more the person who stutters feels the need for greater control of the speaking situation. He may resort to impressing his audience at these times with his "intellectual brilliance," his charm, or the use of witty remarks or to even minimizing his own stuttering in order to win over his listeners. Absolute control of the speaking situation and of his audience helps him maintain some integration and organization when danger arises. Could he now interrupt himself at this precarious point and stop speaking while he still could save face, it would be of some benefit to him. However, the person who stutters seems to gamble only for high stakes in his struggle toward self-idealization. To salvage part of himself, he feels, is not enough. His belief in magical omnipotence is so great that he drives himself in the speaking situation to a state of practical chaos and disorganization. When this occurs, the only alternative left to him is to take flight or to hopelessly resign himself to the outcome of the situation.

The person who stutters feels obligated to and tied down by his audience in the speaking situation. Once he begins to speak he feels coerced and feels that he has to be there against his own will and comply entirely with the wishes and demands of the situation. He struggles not only with the actuality of verbalizing, but also in what ways his listeners will react to him when speaking. While speaking he is driven to fix his attention onto his audience, to study their facial expressions carefully, and to try to decipher every one of their inner thoughts concerning his performance in the speaking situation. His own egocentricity demands this attitude in him as he speaks. Since he cannot stand alone on his own self-evaluation and conviction, he can arrive at some understanding of his own worth and status in the speaking situation only through the opinion and assertions of his listeners. His dire need of winning over his audience and receiving their praise and recognition drives him further to orientate all of his feelings, thoughts, and actions in terms of meeting the satisfaction of his listeners and not in relation to his own opinions or wishes. He needs to control his audience and to keep it intact. When he speaks, he demands absolute attention. No one must leave, lest he become irritable and enraged and so begin to stutter. He feels here that since he makes the sacrifice to give to others in the speaking situation, in spite of his "affliction," others should at least have the decency and patience to sit quietly until he finishes speaking. After he is through with whatever he has to say, he feels temporarily relieved, but soon after enters into another state of confusion and turmoil. Anxiously he may now turn to his audience to wait with apprehension for any of their spontaneous remarks concerning his behavior or what he just spoke about. His own alienation, which grows as a result of a movement away from self-actualization, robs him of the possibility of taking stock of his own role in the speaking situation itself. Though it is quite healthy to want other people's opinions and evaluations of our actions, the person who stutters throws the entire weight of his status, when speaking, on to his audience. His vanity in imaginatively perceiving himself as a wonderful and perfect speaker of necessity compels him to become entirely dependent upon the needs and reactions of the environment about him. Since he feels little of himself at most times, and especially so in the speaking situation, he can come alive only by living vicariously through others.

In the stuttering process, a person not only alienates himself from his real self, but when speaking he also alienates his audience from himself. His detachment, aloofness, callousness, whining, abused feelings, suffering, and the stuttering itself drive his audience away from him. The person who stutters, as much as he stands in awe of others' evaluation of himself in the speaking situation, has also a bitter contempt toward himself and others for having to be so helpless and dependent upon his audience. Unconsciously he will exercise his arrogance and use derogatory remarks to widen the gap between himself and his listeners. The actual stuttering in itself is a means of removing himself from others through its annoying and disturbing quality to those who have to listen. The person who stutters in a sense does not talk to others, but when in control of his speech feels as though he is now the stronger in the situation and can talk down to his audience. The conflict between the desire to be aloof and utterly independent of others and the need to feel completely dependent upon his auditors increases his stuttering.

The stutterer's prime concern when in proximity to others is, first, how is that person going to regard him, rather than how is he going to react to the other person. He feels at most times inferior to others, and this is especially so in the speaking situation, where he feels most threatened. He feels the greatest threat in relation to those people who represent some degree of authority, prestige, or social importance. These people frighten him more than others because they come closest to his own repressed omnipotence and feelings of mastery. He may experience these people as being the most critical, the sternest, or the most demanding as auditors. What actually occurs is that the threat they represent to his particular sensitive personality structure causes him to increase his own perfectionistic expectations upon himself, and thus he feels all the more pressured. Again, since at these times his main regard is to satisfy his auditors, and since he is blind to the fact that these attitudes stem basically from his own inner feelings of inadequacy, the final response can be only one of resentment and bitterness toward those people whom he may feel as causing disruption to his weakened status quo.

A healthy solution can come about when such a disturbed person is able to accept himself as he is and not to drive himself toward self-idealization. Once he becomes less alienated from himself and realizes constructively the shortcomings in his neurotic makeup, he will then be able to take responsibility for whatever he does or says in the speaking situation. Once this responsibility is established, he can perceive his auditors as his equals, and the speaking situation becomes a less threatening one to him.

ATTITUDES TOWARD THE PERSON OR THING DISCUSSED

The person who stutters, in a sense, lives through his own words, including both the spoken and the written word. His words have omnipotent significance to him and move along with his image of being the great talker. His egocentricity compels him to experience objects or things referred to when he speaks as pertaining solely to himself; there is no real audience. Since he has to speak perfectly, he feels in competition with himself and with others. He also feels that he has to use the best descriptive terms, make the most succinct remarks, and have complete understanding or knowledge of whatever he is talking about. To fall short of these expectations in himself makes him feel that he will be rendered vulnerable and prey to his auditors. To have command over himself at all times in the speaking situation is one of the prime ways in which such a person feels he can protect his weakened structure and gain some form of pseudo integration.

The person who stutters exhibits a great sense of dependence upon his words as the sole means of communication for most of his feelings, opinions, and attitudes. He feels that only through words can he make himself understood, and since he is weak in the speaking situation, his whole approach to communication is distorted. This adherence to words is of a strict and rigid quality. Within himself he feels compelled stringently to use the "perfect word," yet at the same time he rebels strongly against any form of outside coercion, be it implicit or explicit. When referring to a thing or an object as he speaks, he gives himself little freedom or choice of words. He is driven to be perfect, exacting, and absolutely correct in all of his communications.

When speaking, he feels driven to know what his position is at all times, not only in reference to himself, but mainly to his auditors and the thing or object he is discussing. This absolute control is felt by him as imperative, since he recognizes how hypersensitive his organism is to the slightest criticism, rebuff, or reversal in the speaking situation. As he refers to an object or thing, he feels threatened whenever he is unable to have this before him or within his immediate grasp. This is especially so because should he have difficulty in using words when referring to a thing or object, he can save face by immediately turning about and pointing to this same thing or object. For instance, a person who stutters has much less difficulty in speaking about a thing or object that is within close proximity to him than those which are distant or intangible. He must always feel in complete control of all objects or things about him. This is especially so when he speaks on the telephone, which he dreads intensely.

To sum up this chapter, the speaking situation controls the major part of the stutterer's feelings, thoughts, and actions. He feels himself caught hopelessly in the grip of this situation. The speaking situation controls him and directs his actions in almost every instance. He does not and cannot feel at these times as "the master of his own ship."

Stuttering, to begin with, is an outward expression of anxiety in conflict, secondary to faulty personality development, and expresses itself specifically and implicitly in the speaking situation. In stuttering, the lines of normal communication are disturbed. Since we tend to think, feel, and act as wholes and not in parts, our speech would of necessity follow the general direction of our inner emotions, attitudes, and beliefs. I would like to refer to the actual process of hesitant and difficult speech as stuttering and to the specific behavioral responses manifested in the stutterer himself at the time he speaks as language behavior. Difficulty in communication per se, I feel, is not the basic problem of the person who stutters. What is more essential is not so much a consideration of the specific words causing trouble at the time a person stutters or a semantic approach to his language structure, but the particular emotional responses that their connotations evoke in the person who is speaking. It is more informative to arrive at a picture of a stutterer's total response to himself and to his listener when he feels anxious and stutters than to know the specific words over which he hesitates. Feared or bugaboo words in stuttering are crucial only in the picture conveyed to us in our attempts to arrive at what is he trying to avoid when he feels endangered and what is felt as threatening to him at the time he is having difficult speech.

To sum up this aspect of the problems, I feel it must be more important, for instance, to comprehend what the stutterer is conveying to us in terms of his innermost feelings and meanings, in any particular speaking situation than why he is using this or that word at the time he stutters. To attempt to understand or treat the person who stutters without an insight into his deeper inner turmoils appears too mechanistic and fixated an approach. To encourage a stutterer to speak up or to speak slowly, whenever he fears he may stutter, alleviates the situation only temporarily. Unless this same person has some deeper understanding of and real feeling for the many compulsive, contradictory tendencies in himself at the time he speaks, no basic reconstruction of his difficulty can possibly come about. He may attempt to control his stuttering by sheer will power, to learn better devices for avoiding bugaboo words, or to speak in a rapid, flighty manner so as to race through the possibility of stuttering before he is through speaking, but all this is automaton-like behavior. I understand there are some persons working with stutterers who even urge them to develop a callousness and boldness toward others in general, the major emphasis being to "fear nothing and care little about others when you speak." This process of consciously undermining the seriousness and the suffering involved in stuttering is a most negative and harmful philosophy. To help himself stutter less, the stutterer must first find and understand himself. Once he has achieved this to some extent, he will feel himself more as a human being with his own convictions, assertions, and personal freedom of thought and expression. The speaking situation at this point is no longer experienced as a threatening situation to him, but one in which he is an equal to others and is free to express whatever he has or wishes to say at will. His anxieties will lessen, and the need to stutter as a whole will lessen proportionately. Finally, at this level of growth, since stuttering does carry with it impressions of past imbedded speech patterns and reflexive habit responses, I feel that speech corrective measures and social interacting methods, such as group therapy, can be valuable adjuncts in the treatment of stuttering.

Speech is considered as our most recently developed and most complex, finely balanced muscular activity. Because of its complicated nature and its numerous nerve areas and muscle groups, which require almost perfect coordination and harmony, it is also an area that is easily prone to disorganization and imperformability during periods of intense emotion. Greene states, "When an individual is in a storm of conflicting emotions, lines of communication are broken and the misdirected nerve messages become delayed or diverted. Most of us at some time or other have experienced the distinctly unpleasant condition of speechlessness due to emotional turmoil. If we realize that the stutterer is in just such a state many times a day, our fundamental problem becomes clear." This language disorganization, which is predominant in people who stutter when under undue stress, is an expression of anxiety in response to some immediate threat to their already weakened personality structure.

Language behavior in stuttering can be understood only if we are able to visualize the stutterer as a completely integrated unit with expressive activity observable in his (overt) behavior, such as talking, walking, sleeping, etc., plus implicit behavior (subjectively experienced), including thinking, feeling, wishing, and understanding. It is the awareness of these total integrated components in action in any given situation that give meaning and direction to his behavior. It is with this holistic approach to behavior in mind that I refer to the stuttering process in the specific speaking situation. It is the total person who stutters in other words and not just one part of him.

In order to arrive at a deeper understanding of the total personality structure of the person who stutters, we must of necessity gain some insight into his language behavior. As he speaks, and especially when he stutters, it is imperative that we be alert enough to attempt to penetrate his inner defenses and approximate some of his hidden feelings and thoughts. As we go behind the scenes of his reactions, including both overt and implicit ones, at the time of heightened anxiety and conflict, we are able to unravel some of the confusions and hidden implications and mysteries implicit in his stuttering. Finally, we must make an attempt to understand not only his objective or externalized speech, but his inner or internalized speech as well.

Impaired communication in speech denotes both interpersonal difficulties, that is disturbances in relation to others and those of an intrapsychic nature, that is disturbances in relation to one's self. In order to comprehend some of the intrapsychic factors in stuttering, I feel it essential that we have some knowledge of the stutterer's symbolic language. Of the later term, Fromm in his book *The Forgotten Language* writes, "Symbolic language is a language in which inner experiences, feelings and thoughts are expressed as if they were sensory experiences, event in the outer world. It is a language which has a different logic from the conventional one we speak in the daytime, a logic in which not time and space are the ruling categories but intensity and association . . . ." An example of symbolic deciphering is the attempt to grasp the full meaning behind such a simple expression from a stutterer as, "I'm stuck with a word. I can't go on talking." At face value, it is meant to express just what it verbally states. That is, the specific individual is having difficulty speaking and can't seem to get past a particular feared or bugaboo word. However, once we get behind the defenses of his character armor, we can arrive at a much deeper understanding of his state of chaos and disorganization. What he now seems to be conveying to us in symbolic fashion is that he basically feels anxious and helpless in the face of overwhelming threats to his neurotic pride and protective defenses. He is also revealing, through language behavior, the threat to his imagined omnipotence in being the perfect speaker at all times who lies in potential failure or disapproval in the speaking situation. Finally, this psychic disunity is externalized to the outside, and what expresses itself overtly is the expression of stuttering, with all its hesitations and blocks. The stuttering individual, once he blocks, feels this blocking and inhibition with his whole personality, resulting in final disturbance of feelings, thinking, and actions.

An understanding of language behavior in stuttering is of crucial importance in the total evaluation and understanding of the stuttering process. We must approach the stutterer as a holistic human being who suffers from emotional difficulties that are expressed overtly when he speaks and especially so at the time of stuttering, if we are to be able to help him find himself and work through his innermost confusions, with all of his anxieties. Only when he finds real inner balance will he achieve healthy coordination of his feelings and actions, including that of relaxed and spontaneous speech.

Chapter 6

TREATMENT IN STUTTERING

IN a problem as complex as stuttering, any attempt toward treatment should be composite in nature. Adequate therapy should include investigations of a medical, social, psychiatric, and reeducational nature. Stuttering is not to be considered as an isolated disorder of the speech mechanism, but as an outward expression of a more basic character disorganization. Any effective treatment must also be directed toward helping the individual understand his particular emotional difficulties, and arrive at some resolution of the underlying conflicts. I shall attempt to describe in as brief and effective a way as possible a therapeutic approach to stuttering that follows the original premises in this book. I hope it may prove workable for the psychiatrist, the speech teacher, the psychologist, allied people in the field of speech disorders, and especially the stutterer himself.

The goals in treatment have changed considerably from those of our forerunners. Today the emphasis is away from symptoms as the prime expressions of underlying disturbances and toward the treatment of the total personality, the whole person. This holistic approach involves not only the individual's disturbances in relation to others, but the nature and importance of intrapsychic processes. Our responsibility is not only to help the stutterer overcome or alleviate his stuttering, but to find himself as an individual and to release those energies now bottled up in his struggle toward self-realization, toward capacities for creative work, better human relationships, and assumption of responsibility for himself.

The belief that stuttering and allied emotional disorders are

best treated with a holistic approach instead of symptomatic relief finds common agreement today. Differences among therapists
lie chiefly in the different foci of emphasis and in the method of
tackling individual character structure. For instance, one common
misconception regards stuttering as originating from a single specific cause, secondary to some emotional traumatic event in the person's past, and that if this can only be uncovered the stuttering
will then disappear. Such thinking was influenced by the early
studies of Freud and his co-workers in their work on hysteria.
From it arises the idea that dramatic cures are possible in stuttering. As a result many stutterers have sought cures of a miraculous
nature for symptomatic removal. Though hypnotism and many
other brief therapeutic approaches do produce an immediate lessening of the speech difficulty, they accomplish little or nothing
in inducing changes in the total personality. A comprehensive
therapeutic approach must focus not only on the early development of the individual but also on basic conflicting tendencies
through all phases of life, with an understanding of both constructive and destructive inhibiting forces. With all of this pertinent
data at hand, therapy may be directed toward a reorientation of
the individual by making available to him whatever constructive
resources are possible toward healthy growth and away from unhealthy development. Once this is accomplished or is in process
of development, we can expect a gradual lessening of anxiety and
an amelioration of the symptom of stuttering itself.

THE THERAPEUTIC PROCESS

A detailed presentation of treatment in stuttering is too
highly specialized a task for one chapter. Only the basic principles
and methods of effective treatment can be summarized here, so
as to give practical help to the speech therapist, the parent, or to
the stutterer himself. Aside from the preventive and educational
procedures that are of value in all disease entities, treatment in
this particular context will be undertaken from a psychiatric or
psychotherapeutic approach. The latter is based on the premise
that stuttering is an emotional problem, resulting from a faulty
development of the individual personality structure.

Despite the fact that in most cases stuttering begins between the ages of two and five, the treatment in American children lies for the most part in the hands of speech therapists in the public schools. Unfortunately, unless a speech therapist is adequately trained in the clinical aspects of stuttering, they may do more harm than good. Doctor Joseph Sheehan, in a 1970 study at the University of California, wrote that "the most conservative conclusion is that our data show that public school therapy of the kind represented in these studies definitely does not facilitate recovery and possibly retard it . . . . Being enrolled in therapy raises hopes, and when nothing results, hopes are dashed, and future motivation is diminished . . . . Moreover, many stutterers acquire an attitude of hopelessness, give up the search, and deny themselves the possibility of future therapy that might really help them."

A successful therapeutic approach to stuttering in the young child must conceive of stuttering as a problem in communication from a psychological viewpoint, as well as the physiological components in the child's struggle with speech. The therapist, whether his training is restricted to speech therapy, psychiatry, psychology, or social work, should have some background and a certain degree of competency in both the psychodynamics of human behavior and the intricacies of speech developments as well as the knowledge of certain specific correctional skills.

Since stuttering usually begins at an early age, treatment too should begin as early as possible. For therapeutic purposes we can distinguish two phases of stuttering: primary and secondary. In treatment during the primary stage (five to ten years of age), when the child is less cognizant of and anxious about his speech problem, the approach is mainly one of treating the parents and, through them, removing unfavorable environmental influences. The prime objective is to be able to give support and yet aid the child to lessen the degree of his inner turmoil and conflicts, to attempt to arrest the disorder, and finally, if possible, to prevent perpetuation of the problem into the secondary stage or into confirmed stuttering. The parents or parent surrogates of the stuttering child are made as aware as possible of the many workable means available to ease the demands made upon their children and how these same pressures can lead to stuttering. An ideal situation, it goes without saying, would be one where either or both of the parents could be encouraged to enter into treatment themselves, to help them work through some of their own most disturbing emotional problems, which in turn would better the child-parent relationship. Where this is not feasible or is met with resistance, treatment of parents must assume the form of specific instructions. These instructions are directed toward (1) improving the general health of the child; (2) balancing his environmental tempo with the removal of some of the more exciting and disturbing tension factors; (3) attempting to encourage in the child a sense of confidence, responsibility, mutual love, and respect; (4) working toward a sense of coordination and rhythm in the child's personality as a whole; (5) encouraging the child to feel free to mix freely with other children and especially with members of his own family; (6) encouraging more constructive methods of discipline; (7) enabling the child to grow at his own particular pace and helping him find his own potentialities and creative capacities; (8) establishing a feeling of real love, warmth, and mutual belonging in the family unit; and, finally, (9) avoiding making the child feel unique or different from others, and especially avoiding making him "speech conscious." In connection with the last-named factor, it is specially urged that the child be allowed to develop a sense of freedom of expression through speech and a feeling for an independent choice of words. Though these goals may seem to be so comprehensive as to be difficult of attainment, even some partial achievement of them can aid the stuttering child in his later struggles toward self-realization.

In the secondary stage of stuttering (eleven to nineteen years of age), the stutterer is now consciously aware that he has a speech difficulty and is particularly affected by what others think of him. This adolescent or adult stutterer develops a keen sensitivity around his affliction of speech and is easily affected by criticism and his own particular shortcomings. The speaking situation now assumes specific colorings of anxiety and apprehensions, which become embedded in his particular character structure. Treatment in this secondary stage of stuttering, in contrast to that of the primary stage, consists primarily of a direct approach. The individual's problems are tackled directly, and the aim is toward personality reorganization. The difference between treating the adolescent and the adult stutterer is mainly qualitative. It is desirable to treat stutterers in this stage also as early as possible, when they are first aware of their problem, since many conflicts are less entrenched and less complex in early adolescence than in later adult years. Also, in the early development phases, patients are more aware of their emotional solutions, which are closer to the surface. They have a greater need and desire to do something about their difficulties, have more available constructive forces, and have less of a neurotic attachment to the symptom of stuttering in itself. Unfortunately, however, the vast majority of stutterers under treatment today are adults. Many of them when children were kept away from treatment through ignorance or blind spots in their parents or else became victims of so-called authorities who advised that they would "outgrow" the disorder. The tragic result was that they discovered too late that they became, instead, chronic stutterers with many more additional conflicting tendencies and a neurotic structure much more difficult to treat.

On the whole, treatment at this stage is usually a combination of psychological, social, and speech therapies. In this context speech therapy is not meant to be of a correctional method, but one that gives symptomatic relief. This should be done by dealing directly with the child's innermost anxieties and fears regarding his speech and can be executed in a simple, clear manner at the child's level. It can be pointed out, for instance, in children with present marked stuttering manifestations, that with relaxation of the muscles of the mouth and neck and with a lowering of the voice, the words come out with no effort. The therapist can demonstrate what actually takes place mechanistically when excessive pressure is put within the mouth area and then can illustrate how easily speech flows when there is no muscular tension. Most children of ten are amazed and appear to be relieved that by following these easy procedures he has no difficulty speaking. Philip J. Glosner, in the chapter "The Psychotherapy of the Young Stutterer" in the book *The Psychotherapy of Stuttering*, edited by Dominick A. Barbara, M.D., wrote, "This approach can be couched in a spirit of play and the child can engage in the activity playing the 'hard' and 'easy' way. This technique tends to take away the mystery or the overwhelming nature of the stuttering . . . . The confidence in the therapy and the relief of anxiety promoted by this technique may be an invaluable wedge into the child's world."

In any successful therapy with the young stutterer, a permissive kind of therapy is usually indicated. In this sense, play therapy is a useful tool. The term *play therapy* includes a multiplicity of activities whose main goal is in developing a positive and warm relationship with the child and a means of understanding his feelings, anxieties, resentments, fantasies, and goals. Play is the child's normal medium of expression, and it allows the therapist to participate in the child's world and to establish a positive transference.

Each therapist must develop his own particular techniques or skills with the child and should utilize the medium and approaches he can handle comfortably. The therapist cannot be rigid and expect to work in the same manner with any two cases. The underlying dynamics are never the same, and therefore, approaches must vary. An effective approach is one that is planned around the needs of the child based upon the therapist's knowledge of the child's problems.

Equation of the Therapist

In dealing with the problem of stuttering, because of its involved and complex nature, the equation of the therapist is of crucial importance. The therapeutic situation is also a human relationship, and whatever difficulties the patient may have in regard to other people operate here too. In order to function at some level of competency, the therapist should have most or some of the following essential requirements:

1. He should have his own personal problems reasonably well solved or be sufficiently well aware of them so that they will not interfere with his working constructively with others.
2. He should be able to handle most eventualities that may occur in the therapeutic situation and be integrated enough to assimilate them without too destructive counterreactions. In this same context, he should be able to handle his own reactive anxieties and hostilities without harming the patient's

progress at the time.

3. He must have an inherent belief in man's ability to change and to grow toward self-realization. He must also have a feeling for process in changing, a knowledge of the patient's fear of it, and the skill to handle defenses against it effectively.

4. He must to some degree be well-oriented in the dynamics of stuttering. In this same area, he should be flexible enough to use as many therapeutic tools as possible that will help toward effecting change.

5. He should have an awareness of and an understanding for the person who stutters. Here, having been a stutterer himself, will be of obvious benefit. He should also have a reading knowledge of the subject of stuttering, its various theories, its working hypothesis, and its present-day methods of treatment.

6. The therapist should be, in every aspect of his personality, a human being. He should have a feeling for struggle and suffering in humans and use every constructive asset in himself toward expressing warmth, understanding, sincerity, and respect for the patient's own wishes and rights. Finding these qualities in the therapist, the patient will have won half the battle: the feeling of mutuality with his therapist, and the understanding the he is at his side, ready to help in most emergencies.

Initial Interview

The initial interview has many important functions. It can be used for diagnostic means, prognostic or therapeutic purposes, and also as a medium to help the patient prepare for the future therapy. The therapist has a challenging responsibility in this particular situation, and many have to make some very important decisions before it is concluded. When in doubt it is wiser to have the patient return for a second or third meeting before making any conclusive decisions, thus avoiding any serious damage to the patient's future therapy.

In the initial meeting with the patient, the therapist is in a strategic position to get his first bird's-eye view of the person who is seeking help. In a strict sense, treatment actually begins here, although there may have been previous contact with the patient by other sources, such as the telephone, a letter, or another person. We learn a great deal about the patient through our first impressions and intuitive feelings. We can also gather pertinent facts about him through our observations of him as he greets us, his manner of approach, his gait, his posture and physical proportions, his smile, his mood, his voice, the color of his eyes, the condition and grooming of his hair, the texture of his skin, the way he wears his clothes, etc. These and so many more manifestations can be utilized in helping us to understand their personality makeup and the possible attitudes and ways in which they experience living.

The initial interview is also a basic source for a number of important facts and data that the therapist must know about his patient before beginning adequate therapy. Briefly, these include name, age, sex, marital status, occupation, religion, education, social status, family background, sibling relations, medical history, early childhood, adolescence and adult development, and sexual history. During this first interview the patient also describes his immediate symptoms and complaints. (In addition, a detailed record of all symptoms and complaints, and primarily that of stuttering, is of prime importance.) The therapist should ask for information pertaining to the age at onset of stuttering, how and where it started, its connection with any traumatic experience or experiences, and when he first began to associate the first objective and subjective feelings of anxiety with his speech defect. In this same orientation, it is important to seek data concerning a specific familial history of stuttering, parental attitudes toward his speaking and toward his speech defect, and most essential of all, the patient's own feelings and attitudes about his stuttering throughout his remembered development. Finally, for a more complete picture, it is necessary to have some understanding of the patient's present attitudes about his speech impediment and especially how he experiences himself with it in relation to himself and others. We can now arrive at some beginning working premise of the patient's predominant conflicts, the extent to which he uses his stuttering as a device, and finally some insight into the degree of alienation present.

It goes without saying that since we are treating the personality as a whole and not the symptom of stuttering in itself, we need to gather as much information as possible regarding the patient himself as a living human being, including both intrapsychic and interpersonal factors. In this sense we may question him about his ways of life, his habits, his likes and dislikes, his preference for others, his capacities, abilities, potentialities, and something about his dreams, fantasies, and imagination. As he speaks, we can also arrive at some of his possible reactions to ourselves as therapists, the manner in which he may attempt to avoid direct answers, the use of bugaboo words, or means of rituals and distractions when he feels he may be about to stutter. These and kindred points of observation are some of the unlimited resources we have at hand in the first few initial interviews, which can be of tremendous importance as we proceed with the therapeutic process.

Before the therapist can plan any direct plan of approach, it is essential that he pull together all these facts and personal observations and make some of his own concluding impressions. At this point he must evaluate to the best of his judgment and therapeutic acumen the following essential basic criteria:

1. The relative degree of constructive assets and real incentives for help present in the patient in relation to opposing negative and retarding forces. Also from what sources at hand and from those more hidden can we look for and make available energies toward self-realization.
2. The degree and extent of alienation.
3. The patient's extent of awareness of his own problems, his real desires for help, the feeling for change, and finally his capacity for cooperation in the therapeutic situation.
4. The degree of severity of his obvious symptoms and primarily that of his stuttering.
5. Finally, a measure of the patient's awareness of and capacity for struggle, a sense for real suffering, and his threshold for anxiety.

Working with Resistances

Once the primary objectives are established and a plan of approach is decided upon by the therapist, then more feasible and productive therapeutic work can begin. In accordance with the original premises of this book, especially that of promoting self-realization, it is important to recognize early in the therapeutic process the various resistances and blockages that are keeping the stuttering process going and simultaneously are interfering with healthy growth. Since we are primarily interested in helping the patient find himself, we must remove those obstacles that obstruct his growth, interfere with his real self, and cause him to feel alien to himself and to others.

In order to keep the therapeutic process alive and moving, the therapist should be as real and spontaneous a person as possible himself. He should be concerned primarily with the patient's capacity for withstanding anxiety rather than with his own personal success, failure, or reactivating inner disturbances. He should have a spirit of mutuality, and the quality of his attention and interpretations should be sincere, human, truthful, and democratic in nature. He should understand that the patient is attempting to hold onto his way of life, with all its unhealthy solutions, because he is convinced within himself of its worth and because these solutions give him a sense of unity without which he might endanger his whole psychic equilibrium.

In people who stutter there is present a great deal of pride invested in the irrational claims they make upon themselves and others. This area presents tremendous resistance to change. To help the stutterer feel that he is not necessarily a cripple because he has difficult speech at times, and therefore is not entitled to any special privileges from others, is a problem most difficult to tackle. This sort of compulsive behavior comes from two basic sources: from a feeling of being victimized and abused since early childhood and from an imaginative concept of themselves as "chosen people," privileged in every aspect of living.

Unless other factors in the therapeutic situation warrant immediate attention, I feel that this wide area of claims should be tackled immediately or as soon as feasible. Once the stutterer develops some feeling of rapport and a sense of confidence with this therapist and has gained supportive ground to stand on, he should be helped to face this problem of claims. This whole area, with its many ramifications, interactions, and consequences, needs to be laid open and worked through before the therapeutic process as a whole can move forward constructively.

It is impossible to describe in one brief chapter the numerous technical problems that can arise in attempting to expose these claims. I can only say that the therapist, utilizing as human and helpful an approach as possible, must attempt to undermine the special neurotic prides invested in the particular claims brought to discussion by showing the patient, through valid concrete examples, the irrationality of his demands. He can also bring to light the rigid characteristics of the reasoning behind these claims. He can help the patient to understand that these claims are based predominantly on imaginary merits rather than actual or potential worth. Finally, the patient must arrive at an understanding of the many interacting operating forces behind his claims, the intensity of the drivenness and it compulsive qualities, and most essential of all, his particular role in actively perpetuating its machinery. Once the patient gains some insight into the retarding nature of these claims, and especially of those used in the speaking situation, he will feel less coerced and consequently more hopeful and courageous about his whole future treatment.

Areas Where Blockages Are Predominant

Difficulties Shown Before Starting Treatment. *A major problem in the treatment of stuttering is how to encourage the stutterer to stay in and continue with the course of treatment.* First of all, this, of course, involves an evaluation of the real incentives in the individual patient and what his specific expectations will be once he consents to starting therapy.

Since many stutterers may have gone from clinic to clinic, consulted with various specialists, or in the case of the more unfortunate ones, been subjected to so-called *miraculous cures*, some doubts and feelings of doom and hopelessness will have become fixed. As a result, when they are initially interviewed for what they may feel to be another new and futile attempt, among the many others, they are often skeptical and cautious and may by this time have little real incentive for receiving help toward solving their problems. It is in relation to this difficult area of resistance that the therapist must give a great deal of himself by way of courageousness. He might begin by giving the patient some pertinent data about his own professional background and experiences with psychological problems, especially with the specific problem of stuttering. He should try to help alleviate the patient's doubts about himself and some of his anxiety by putting him at ease and relating to him in a firm but sincere, warm, open, and consistent manner. He can further reassure the patient with remarks such as, "Yes, I have no doubts about being able to help you with your problems, provided you are ready to cooperate with me, and help pitch in so that we can do the job together."

It is especially important that the therapist should not make promises that he does not intend to or cannot fulfill later on. Not only are false promises dishonest; they can lead to catastrophic difficulties in the course of treatment and may even end in the patient's leaving therapy in a more despairing and disbelieving state of mind than the one in which he entered it. The real facts about his illness and the degree of severity of his complaints (providing they can be presented to the patient without shaking too strongly his already weakened foundation) should be revealed to him so that he can get a realistic perspective. This may temporarily jar the patient's neurotic status quo, but in the long run it will add to his feelings of respect and sense of mutuality toward the therapist.

Blockages in Patient's Productivity. Aside from the usual hesitations found in the stutterer's way of speaking, there are present similar inhibitions and blocks in the quality of his productions. In fact, the person who stutters blocks with his whole organism, including his feelings, attitudes, beliefs, and actions.

As has been stated previously, the stutterer takes a great deal of pride in wisdom and intellect. He thinks in terms of absolutes, and many of his responses are purely at an intellectual level. His own inner fear of feelings compels him to seek for logical and clean-cut answers to his problems. In his attempts to seek his conflicts at a distance, he attempts to compartmentalize and rationalize many of his shortcomings and opposing tendencies.

The stutterer's associations are usually not free and spontaneous in quality. Since this interferes with the progress of treatment, it is imperative that the patient be educated and made aware of this blocking agent early in treatment in order to promote a more real and down-to-earth atmosphere in the therapeutic situation it-self. He may bring to his interview an abundance of material, yet it may be of such a reportorial nature that it can have very little real meaning to his actual feelings or conflicts. The therapist should be constantly on the alert for this sort of underproductive activity because it can be deceiving. He should help the patient to look "behind the scenes" of his productions, in order to discover whatever special meanings his associations may convey to his own particular needs, feelings, and motivations at the time of expression. Material that is remote to the patient and felt at a distance to his inner core or felt as if coming from somewhere outside of him leaves very little impression on the patient and brings about little constructive insight. To help the patient at this point to be eager to talk about himself and be interested in his own welfare is of great importance.

Among blockages in productivity is, of course, that of the actual stuttering symptom. If a therapist is not thinking of working with the total character structure, he can easily involve himself in a hopeless struggle toward removing the symptom itself. With such an approach, he can easily get caught in a confusing entanglement of intellectual discussions centering mainly around presupposed cause-and-effect correlations of stuttering, losing meanwhile the background of the whole person. It is important to keep in mind what the stutterer is trying to express each time he speaks, primarily when he is stuttering. The way he presents himself when he speaks, with his many hidden meanings, feeling tones, anxieties, inhibitions, hesitations, and especially his own word jargon, is highly connotative of himself, providing we are there to intercept and decode the message. A whole volume could be written on this subject.

Disturbances in the Therapist-Patient Relationship. The therapist-patient relationship is a human relationship like all others and of special significance as a milieu where establishing good rapport can lead toward self-realization. There are, however, qualitative differences concerning the relative positions: The therapist is the more trained and experienced in psychological problems, while the patient who comes for help may look up to the therapist as an authority.

Problems found in every other human relationship are just as prevalent in the therapeutic relationship. For instance, the person who stutters makes the same claims on the therapist that he may make upon others, and this tends ultimately to hinder the therapeutic progress. His glorified self strives for absolute productivity. He meets reversals with despair and hopelessness. He feels obliged to find a rapid solution to his conflicts without sincere motive or realistic effort. From his therapist he may demand not only perfection but also immediate, absolute attention at all times. He may expect the therapist to make more frequent interpretations and to work with him more actively. But at the same time he becomes very antagonistic and resistant toward making any compromises or sacrifices himself; he feels that his mere presence entitles him to change.

His fantastic notions and claims gradually force his submission to the tyranny of the should, and he begins to have a sense of doom and a feeling of helplessness. His failure to progress rapidly and to sense a more constructive and positive inner change leads to a further state of inner coercion and feelings of hopelessness. He pushes himself up blind alleys and finally must appeal to the mercy of his therapist to lift him from the abyss of self-contempt and misery. The expectations on the part of the patient are in the beginning phases of treatment mainly of an irrational nature. He will attempt to look for discrepancies in his therapist and will appeal to neurotic residuals in him, rather than the human side. In order to uphold his own protective structure, the patient may resort to every possible form of stratagem in order to confuse, defeat, humiliate, or "show up" his therapist. He may try to keep the therapist at a distance with arrogance or aloofness, to manipulate him, or to even attempt to become chummy or to reduce him with charm. If any of these maneuvers, which are attempts to keep conflicts out of awareness, do not achieve their objective, he may then feel attacked and be constantly on the defensive. This latter situation is especially felt when the individual's pride is undermined, and his vital existence is endangered and experienced as threatening. It is in this stormy and delicate part of the therapeutic relationship that the patient must feel and communicate to his therapist as a friend and one whom he feels to be both confidential and trustworthy. If such a feeling of interrelatedness and mutuality can be accomplished and further developed by both therapist and patient, then the patient can feel less frightened and will have more courage to search within himself for further constructiveness.

Another formidable obstructing force in the therapeutic relationship is that of the patient's use of magical claims. He externalizes his own feelings of magic onto the therapist and endows him with special superhuman powers impossible to attain. He feels that his therapist should be a magician who can, without the slightest effort, pull him out of his dilemma. The person who stutters may use his stuttering with all of its distractions and rituals as a powerful means of keeping his therapist off guard and thus in a less threatening position to his inner stability. It is of utmost importance for the therapist to maintain a balanced, firm, and consistent position in spite of the patient's attempts to keep him off guard and in an inferior status. Though the patient may appear to battle firmness or consistency in the therapist, he secretly and basically desires it. It will ultimately give him a sense of security and a feeling of real respect and regard for his therapist.

Maintenance of the Neurotic Status Quo. The stutterer's fear of change and his tenacious defense of positions that give him a sense of pseudo unity offer other areas of resistance and blockage in the therapeutic process. This attempt at maintaining the status quo protects anxiety to some extent and gives him a false set of values with which he can exist without too much psychic disorganization and, lastly, provides for defenses in maintaining his illusions of himself.

The person who stutters is in constant fear and dread of having his protective structures invaded or removed because of the accompanying terror of crumbling and psychically "going to pieces." His constant need for mastery, especially in the speaking situation, causes him to generate feelings of self-hate whenever his pride values in this direction are undermined. Unable to face his conflicts squarely or to bear their accompanying anxiety, he is prone to fall back too quickly on old defense measures in pleading helplessness and having abused feelings. The more desperate he feels his situation to be, the greater the number of strategies needed to cope with his endangered position. His last area of retreat, at least in his way of thinking, is finally that of avoiding conflict altogether by resigning himself to a state of pseudo unity, thus being able to save face in at least part of the struggle.

As the stutterer desperately attempts to hold onto his "status quo," the therapist must not add to the struggle by hitting back, forcibly pulling against him, or trying to impress him with his superior intellect. The problem is not just one of digging the stutterer out of his entrenched position, but of coming to an understanding of his role in the particular conflicting situation. By helping him to look at the possible reasons behind his fear of letting go of old protective defenses, and more specifically what he feels he is warding off, he can now slowly come to a realistic understanding of his struggle between self-idealization and self-realization.

It is essential that the person who stutters begins to see himself less as just a stutterer and to have more feelings for himself as a human being, in spite of his stuttering. Once he is encouraged to feel less hopeless, resigned, and frustrated, the more firm ground can be feel himself to stand on. As a result, he will feel less threatened from his weakened position, feel less anxious, and then have the courage to face himself as he really is, to take a stand in relation to his conflicts, and to have courage to change.

End Stages of Treatment

So far, what has been said concerning the undermining of the pride system and the working with resistances and blockages is in essence a disillusioning process. However, they alone, as Horney states, "could not and would not have a thorough and lasting liberating effect (if any) if constructive moves did not set in simultaneously.

"The therapeutic value of the disillusioning process lies in the possibility that, with the weakening of the obstructive forces, the constructive forces of the real self have a chance to grow."

Since healing forces are present in the patient from the very beginning, it is essential to start mobilizing these constructive assets at the very onset of therapy. Later on, as he moves further away from the periphery of his conflicts and begins to get closer to himself, we may find less of an oblivious reaction to his remoteness from himself and more of an awareness and interest concerning his real feelings, wishes, and beliefs. His alienation becomes lessened, and the patient now becomes interested in the question, "Who am I?" With this growing sense of wisdom about himself, he begins to question many of his present attitudes, feelings, and beliefs and to reevaluate them in the light of reality-tested aspects and with his own inner volition and beginning independence.

The patient at this time also begins to feel himself on more solid ground and more capable of grappling with his conflicts. With less alienation from himself, he will tend less to externalize and rationalize his problems onto the outside, but to experience them instead as coming from somewhere within himself. In the final analysis, the patient is now capable of tackling more directly the most comprehensive conflict of all—to quote Horney: "that between his pride system and his real self, between his drive to perfect his idealized image and his desire to develop his given potentials as a human being."

The final struggle between self-idealization and self-realization can be of a turbulent and violent nature. As the central inner conflict comes more directly into focus, the opposing forces of the dilemma begin to gradually line up and ready themselves for battle. The greater the number of inhibiting forces, the more intense the nature of the struggle will present itself, and conversely. In this same period we will also find a greater number of ups and downs occurring often in rapid succession. The more the patient will attempt to move forward and become more alive or spontaneous, the greater the repercussions from the unhealthy side in the form of self-hate and self-contempt. This same crucial period of self-growth may be characterized by intense feelings of terror and panic on the part of the patient. It is of basic necessity during this shaky period that the therapist give his utmost attention, understanding, and encouragement to the patient's sufferings. He must also be able to respect the patient's tolerance for anxiety and his dire need to hold on "for dear life" to his remaining neurotic protective devices. The therapist who cannot feel for the struggle going on in his patient, who may be too detached, aloof, or objective, or who is interested primarily in his own ambitious success in the therapeutic process can do irreparable damage in this phase of therapy. It sometimes happens at this stage that a patient suddenly turns against his therapist and lashes at him with vindictive rage and hostility. The therapeutic relationship can be so damaged and disturbed that it may be essential to terminate it or to suggest a change in therapist.

As the battle in the struggle toward self-realization comes under control and is finally won, the greatest constructive forces now become available to the individual patient. He can now assume responsibility for his own way of life, give up many of his fictitious values, and discard his illusions about himself. Finally, with more feeling insight into his problems and a lessening of alienation from himself, we find a greater impetus toward self-realization, accompanied by a basic change in values, a new way of life, and more realistic goals.

As the struggle toward self-realization proceeds, there is also a gradual lessening or removal of the symptom of stuttering in itself. As the patient slowly frees himself from the chains of his stuttering, so will be become less driven, compulsive, and indiscriminate in his entity. In the process of changing many aspects of his personality structure, he will also come to understand the various needs, with all their ramifications, interconnections, and consequences, behind his stuttering speech. As he blocks less as a total individual and becomes less inhibited and more flexible as a whole, so will he simultaneously come less often to hesitate and block in his speech.

In the growth toward self-realization, with its healthy reevaluation and reorientation of values and attitudes in many life situations, there will be similar changes in the speaking situation. The stutterer can now feel less inclined to depend morbidly on the opinions of others, to have a greater sense of his own self-worth, and to take more responsibility for himself, even when he speaks. He will learn to feel and experience his words and expressions as his own, coming from within himself, and will have the courage to stand behind his own individual assertions and convictions. The more inner strength he feels, the more solid ground will he feel beneath him and the less inadequate will he present himself in all circumstances, including that of verbal communication. Finally, as he accepts himself more, with or without his stuttering, so will the need to cover up and hide discrepancies become lessened. As he comes out more into the open and assumes a more honest front, he will as a result have much less need to stutter.

Dreams

In dreams, we possess a most valuable tool for helping pave the way toward greater self-understanding and growth. Dreams aid in removing many of our conscious defensive barriers and allow us to move closer to ourselves. Dreams reflect in a most accurate and truthful sense the reality of ourselves, the kinds of conflicts we are experiencing, and the various attempts we use to solve them. Finally, dreams help us to reveal our destructive as well as our constructive impulses in a most clear, specific, precise, and simple manner. Dreams also have the unique and distinct quality of abstracting, crystallizing, and vividly demonstrating hidden aspects of ourselves. They are our own individual creations of ourselves, and in it the patient can visualize his true inner feelings and peculiarities in contrast to the world of his illusions.

Dreams occur in the sleeping state, when we are withdrawn from our more external world with all its conscious pressures and demands. In the dream state we are in closer proximity to our real selves and concurrently feel we can be ourselves more freely. In our dreams there is a greater tendency to be frank and honest with ourselves, to face ourselves more squarely, and to be more able to take stock of our shortcomings and difficulties. Our feelings in dreams, whether pleasant or disturbed, are not disguised and usually are present in their true states. Dreams often tell us of how we stand in relation to our problems, with the actual coloring of our inner emotions.

The various constructive changes that occur in a particular individual's growth can be reflected in a series of recurrent-type dreams or in those dreams in which there are basic connecting similarities. For instance, a stutterer who presented predominantly self-effacing trends had the following recurrent dream early in his treatment: He would dream of himself in a large auditorium, either on stage, about to walk up to a platform, or in front of a microphone ready to deliver a speech. Yet each time at the point of opening his mouth or beginning to utter a sound, he found he couldn't speak, became paralyzed with terror, and would awaken in a cold sweat, palpitating, and out of breath. Later in therapy, when he had made progress and was able to face more of his conflicts, the context of the dream changed to the following: To use the patient's own words, "The dream starts once again with my being in a room. However, this time it isn't the old auditorium with its vastness and cold atmosphere. It is smaller, somewhat familiar and comfortable. Instead of my walking to the platform to speak, I find myself in a group with people who are friendly and congenial. We suddenly all begin to talk in unison. At one point, the conversation ceases, and I find myself speaking alone and directly to the others. What I said, I can't remember, except that I felt calm within myself and didn't have the old panicky feelings. I awoke feeling good." The dream in a sense is self-explanatory. Briefly, it clearly represents this individual's struggle away from self-idealization and toward his real self. The courage to give up his illusions of himself as a great orator with all of its accompanying anxieties, frustrations, and self-hate, is indicated in the moves away from that of self-glorification to that of a more solid and realistic level.

Dreams are also valid indicators of our true inner behavioristic patterns. The stutterer, for instance, is a chronic blocker and hesitator in both the waking and sleeping states. It is not uncommon to find that in his dreams many of his activities and other forms of expression, including that of speaking, become symbolically illustrated with all of their inhibitions and blockages. For instance, a patient of mine who stuttered found that most of his dream sequences were never completed because of numerous unexpected interruptions, such as fires, riots, explosions, and other unforeseen eventualities. His dreams also indicated the intense feelings of indecisiveness, procrastination, and self-doubts, which were part of his total personality structure. In the treatment of stutterers, with all their rigid defenses and impenetrable protective structures, dream examples of this sort are valuable aids in developing a clearer understanding into their problems.

Constructive changes are also symbolized in those dreams that deal with the therapeutic relationship. In his dreams the patient will usually indicate his feelings, attitudes, and perspectives toward his therapist, both rational and irrational. As the course of the treatment progresses and changes, so will the patient's perspectives toward the therapist, gradually progressing through lesser irrationality to greater actuality.

The skill to utilize and work with dreams in the therapeutic situation is of decisive importance in the search for hidden constructive forces in our patients. Our patients will thereby indicate these forces present in themselves. It is our job as therapists to help open passages in their roadblocks so that they can free themselves sufficiently to utilize such constructive forces in their struggle toward self-realization.

Group Therapy

The use of group therapy is a valuable adjunct in the treatment of stuttering. It is of greatest significance when used along with and interchangeably with individual therapy. Alone it would not be as effective. When individual psychotherapy can help the stutterer arrive at an understanding of his more deeply rooted conflicts, the additional use of group therapy will give him the advantage of experiencing himself in social situations, especially in the speaking situation.

The aim of the group approach in the treatment of stuttering is threefold:

1. To break down the stutterer's old, unsound emotional reactions, habit patterns, and attitudes and to help him build up healthy, constructive new ones.
2. To overcome the patient's specific fears and anxieties, especially regarding speech situations.
3. To foster a better social adjustment and to develop a more mature, adequate, and better-integrated personality as a whole.

Following are some of the suggested ways in which the group can help in arriving at their therapeutic objectives:

1. The group creates a situation in which the individual is brought face to face with himself and experiences himself as he really is. It also gives him an opportunity to act against his symptom in the specific situation that ordinarily provokes it.
2. If the group is homogeneous to some degree, it helps him to see that others have similar difficulties, conflicts, and general

personality traits and that he is not alone in his troubled situation. This important subjective feeling of being "in the same boat" with others ultimately adds to his own self-growth. In the case of stutterers, it gives them the valuable experience and opportunity of seeing other people stutter and of learning from their difficulties.

3. In the group situation, the patient is more willing to accept his own limitations and discrepancies when he realizes that he shares them with others. It also helps him to move closer to those others in the group and to improve, in general, his relations to others.

4. The group enables the patient to express himself as freely as possible without inhibition or censorship. In so doing he can gain valuable insight into many of his defenses, prejudices, illusions, blind spots, and various aspects of his speech difficulty. The group situation can be used as a proving ground for testing the validity and reliability of inner feelings and constructive changes in himself as he progresses in individual treatment.

5. The group milieu gives the therapist a real life situation in which to observe his patient with his various attitudes, feelings, and beliefs, especially as these factors operate in relation to others. Material of this sort is of significant importance for discussion and elaboration in those instances where the patient may be simultaneously undergoing individual treatment.

6. In group therapy, the actual disillusioning process, which can be of a very painful nature in individual therapy with all of its tensions and anxieties, is better tolerated by the patient because of the spirit of group acceptance and support.

7. Finally, in those patients where resistance to change is met, the individual is much more likely to remain in therapy when he is part of a group and when he sees the progress others may be making in treatment. It also gives him a realistic awareness of struggle, real suffering, and the need for sacrifices in the process toward growth.

A PROPOSAL FOR A COMBINED
FORM OF THERAPY IN STUTTERING

If speech therapy is to continue its development and to serve more efficiently the needs of the stutterer, the therapist must consider how it is related to the broader areas of the social sciences. This will serve to eliminate a mechanistic approach and to move the speech therapist closer to a wider and fuller holistic entity, connecting him intimately to the field of personality and human development.

In summary and conclusion, my wishes for a joint and combined approach to stuttering can be best summarized by quoting once more from Doctor Jesse J. Villaireal.

In brief summary, the viewpoint presented here includes the following points:

1. Stuttering is more than a speech problem (as most speech problems are) in the sense that it involves more than a deviate way of operating the vocal mechanism.

2. A significant dimension of stuttering, calling for therapeutic attention, is an area of emotional disturbance. Whether this emotional disturbance is viewed as the basic cause of stuttering or the inevitable result of it, makes little difference to the present argument. What is important is that it is there and needs attention.

3. At the same time that it is recognized that stuttering involves more than the manipulation of the vocal mechanism, it is also recognized that it does involve kinds of disorganization that require modifications in the activity of the vocal mechanism, and these areas are those of the speech pathologist.

4. It is therefore necessary, for the most adequate treatment of stuttering, that a therapy team involving both the skills of the speech pathologist and those of the psychotherapist be employed.

5. The efficient functioning of a therapy team in which the speech pathologist and the psychotherapist function cooperatively calls for a familiarity by each specialty of the other. No effort has been made here to spell out in detail the courses and the clock hours of clinical practice by which this mutual awareness may best be guaranteed, but it is obvious that not every speech pathologist is equipped at present to be of aid to the psychotherapist, and the reverse is just as evident.

BIBLIOGRAPHY

Blanton, Smiley, and Blanton, M.D.: *For Stutterers*. New York, D. Appleton-Century Company, 1936.

Bluemel, C.S.: *Stammering and Allied Disorders*. New York, The Macmillan Company, 1935.

Fromm, Erich: *The Forgotten Language*. New York, Rinehard & Company, 1951.

Goldstein, K.: Language and Language Disturbances: *Aphasic Symptom Complexes and Their Significance for Medicine and Theory of Language*. New York, Grune & Stratton, 1948.

Gottlober, A.B.: *Understanding Stuttering*. New York, Grune & Stratton, 1953.

Horney, Karen: *Neurosis and Human Growth*. New York, W.W. Norton & Company, Inc., 1950.

——*The Neurotic Personality of Our Time*. New York, W.W. Norton & Company, Inc., 1947.

——*New Ways in Psychoanalysis*. New York, W.W. Norton & Company, Inc., 1938.

——*Our Inner Conflicts*. New York, W.W. Norton & Company, Inc., 1945.

——*Self-Analysis*. New York, W.W. Norton & Company, Inc., 1942.

Kanner, Leo: *Child Psychiatry*. Springfield, Illinois, Charles C Thomas, 1942.

Meerloo, Joost A.M.: *Conversation and Communication*. New York, International Universities Press, 1952.

Murray, Elwood: *The Speech Personality*. Philadelphia, J.B. Lippincott Company, 1944.

Van Riper, C.: *Speech Correction*. New York, Prentice-Hall, Inc., 1939.

Villarreal, Jesse J.: The role of the speech pathologist in psychotherapy. In Dominick A. Barbara (Ed), *The Psychotherapy of Stuttering*. Springfield, Illinois, Charles C Thomas, 1962.